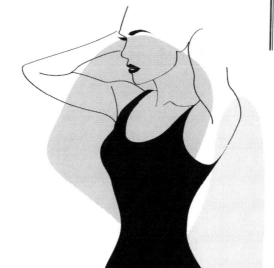

INTERMITTENT FASTING FOR WOMEN OVER 50

Your Complete Beginner's Guide to Burning Fat and Lose Weight Rapidly. Delicious Illustrated Recipes to Reset Metabolism and Detox Your Body.

Carola Taylor

© Copyright 2021 by Carola Taylor - All rights reserved.

The following Book is reproduced below with the goal of providing information that is as accurate and reliable as possible. Regardless, purchasing this Book can be seen as consent to the fact that both the publisher and the author of this book are in no way experts on the topics discussed within and that any recommendations or suggestions that are made herein are for entertainment purposes only. Professionals should be consulted as needed prior to undertaking any of the action endorsed herein.

This declaration is deemed fair and valid by both the American Bar Association and the Committee of Publishers Association and is legally binding throughout the United States.

Furthermore, the transmission, duplication, or reproduction of any of the following work including specific information will be considered an illegal act irrespective of if it is done electronically or in print. This extends to creating a secondary or tertiary copy of the work or a recorded copy and is only allowed with the express written consent from the Publisher. All additional right reserved.

The information in the following pages is broadly considered a truthful and accurate account of facts and as such, any inattention, use, or misuse of the information in question by the reader will render any resulting actions solely under their purview. There are no scenarios in which the publisher or the original author of this work can be in any fashion deemed liable for any hardship or damages that may befall them after undertaking information described herein.

Additionally, the information in the following pages is intended only for informational purposes and should thus be thought of as universal. As befitting its nature, it is presented without assurance regarding its prolonged validity or interim quality. Trademarks that are mentioned are done without written consent and can in no way be considered an endorsement from the trademark holder.

Table of Contents

Introduction	1
What Is Intermittent Fasting	2
Types of Intermittent Fasting	5
Health Benefits of Intermittent Fasting	11
Insider Tips for Breaking a Fast	16
Proven Tips for Managing Your Fast	20
Breakfast for Your Intermittent Fast	25
A Bit of Lunch Cuisine in Between	47
Dinner Meals After the Fast	70
Snacks, Sides, and Salads for Fasting	95
Unique Desserts Your Fast	104
Conclusion	123

INTRODUCTION

Fasting intermittently is not a diet. It's an eating habit and a lifestyle. It's a way to prepare the meals to ensure that one gets the best out of them. Fasting Intermittently doesn't affect what you consume. It matters when you consume food. Intermittent fasting is not only a method for weight reduction or a hack that athletes use to lose fat while easily keeping lean muscle mass. It is a balanced lifestyle influenced by human evolution and the research on metabolism at its finest. Intermittent fasting needs the body to be more self-productive and effective for it to work. Intermittent fasting typically implies that, your intake the calories at a specific time and choose not to eat food for a longer time. Many researches indicates that this form of living can provide benefits such as weight reduction, improved fitness, and enhanced lifespan. Experts claim that it's simpler to sustain an extended fasting regimen than conventional, calorie-controlled diets. Understanding the intermittent fasting of each person is different, and varying types will fit other individuals based on their needs.

Fasting intermittently is one of the best methods people have for reducing excess weight off but holding healthy weight on, and it needs relatively least behavior modification. This is a positive idea because it ensures intermittent fasting fits under the easy enough task that one will simply do it, however significant enough that it can make a transformation. Intermittent fasting shifts hormone levels to promote weight reduction.

In addition to reducing insulin in the bloodstream and increasing growth hormone levels, it enhances the production of the burning fat hormone known as noradrenaline or norepinephrine.

Studies suggest that a very effective method for weight reduction may be intermittent fasting. Short-term fasting can raise the body's metabolic rate by 3.6 to 14 percent due to these hormones' changes. By encouraging one to eat less, burn additional calories, by manipulating all calorie calculation aspects, intermittent fasting induces weight loss.

In contrast to other weight loss trials, a study showed that this eating style would induce 3 to 8 percent weight loss from 3 to 24 weeks, which is a significant change. There is no each-size-fits-all approach when it comes to intermittent fasting at the end of the day. The one approach that you should hold on to in the long term is the right pattern with proper nutrition for you.

The reduction in muscle protein blend is only one reason why the six meals a day program is flawed. Another imperfection is the effect that frequent meals have on your body's capacity to consume fat, which is a significant one for bodybuilders and for people whose goal is to get slender. Providing your body with a consistent inventory of energy supply implies that it will not have to consume fat.

The six meals a day program is based partially on the idea that you will feel less hungry between meals, making you more reluctant to gorge each time you do eat and less inclined to nibble on unhealthy foods between meals. Nevertheless, this can likewise fail much of the time.

People who get one high-protein meal instead of five little meals generally feel less craving later on and eat less at their next meal. This frequent meal advice may make you bound to consume extra calories, which is something opposing to the expected effect of diminishing your hunger.

For certain individuals, intermittent fasting is fine, just not for others. Although, in particular, older people over 50 and women may try it comfortably. Trying it out is the best way to figure out which group you relate to. It can be an effective method to lose weight and boost your wellbeing if you feel comfortable while fasting and believe it to be a sustainable form of eating.

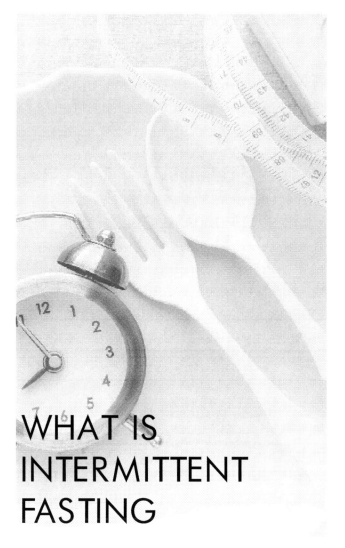

WHAT IS INTERMITTENT FASTING

During intermittent fasting, you would not be pressured to deprive yourself throughout the day, also mentioned as IF. It also doesn't grant you a license during the period of non-fasting to eat loads of unhealthy food. You consume within a fixed window of time, instead of consuming meals and treats all day. Intermittent fasting is an eating pattern model that requires daily, short-term fasts or limited or no food intake at times.

Most individuals know intermittent fasting as losing weight assistance. Intermittent fasting is a lifestyle that allows people to consume fewer calories, leading to weight loss over time.

Without being on an insane diet or consuming the calories to nil, it's a perfect way to get healthy.

Most of the time, when one begins intermittent fasting, they'll aim to maintain their calories the same as during a shortened time; most people consume larger meals. In comparison, prolonged fasting is a healthy way to preserve body mass while becoming lean. But most notably, intermittent fasting is among the most beneficial way to be in shape with many other benefits. This is an easy way to get the desired results. If performed properly, intermittent fasting will have valuable advantages, like weight reduction, type 2 diabetes reversal, and several other aspects. Plus, this will save time and resources for you.

Intermittent fasting is successful because it makes it possible for the amount of insulin and blood sugar to reach a low level. The body's fat-storing enzyme is insulin. Fat moves into the fat cells and gets absorbed when insulin levels are high in the blood; if insulin level is low, fat will move and burn out of fat cells. In short, IF is when food is readily available, but you prefer not to consume it. This may be over any period of time, from several hours to a couple of days, or sometimes a week or more under strict medical monitoring. You can begin fasting at any moment of your choice, and you can end a fast at your will, too.

You fast intermittently if you don't consume food by choice. For instance, between dinner and breakfast, till the following day, you will not eat and fast for around 12 to 14 hours. Intermittent fasting can, in that way, be deemed a part of daily life.

THE SCIENCE BEHIND IT

Like any idea of eating that quickly takes over health and diet cultures, intermittent fasting has been suspected to be a fad. Still, the evidence behind fasting's advantages is already clear— and increasing.

There are several hypotheses as to why intermittent fasting performs so well, but tension has to do with the most widely studied — and most proven gain.

The term stress has been vilified continuously, but the body profits from some stress. Exercise, for example, is technically stress on the body (especially on the muscles and the cardiovascular system). Still, this specific stress ultimately makes the body better as long as you implement the correct amount of recovery period into your exercise plan.

Intermittent fasting stresses the body in the same way that exercise does; it brings the cells under moderate tension as you refuse the body food for a certain period. Cells respond to this tension over time by studying how to better cope with it. It has an improved ability to resist illness because the body becomes better at dealing with pain.

TYPES OF INTERMITTENT FASTING

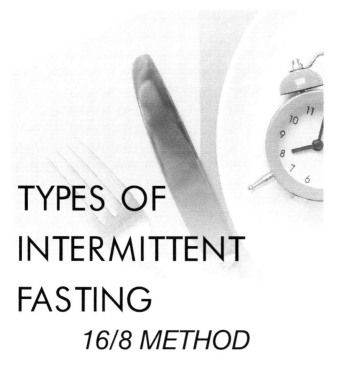

16/8 METHOD

This is just about the most popular fasting methods since it's so schedule based, meaning there are no surprises. This will give you the freedom to control when you eat based on the everyday life of yours. The sixteen is the number of hours you're likely to be fasting, which may also be lowered to twelve or perhaps fourteen hours if that fits into your life better. Then you're eating period is going to be between eight and ten hours every day. This might seem daunting, but it just means that you are skipping an entire meal.

Many people choose to begin their fast around 7 or 8 p.m. and then do not eat until 11 or noon the next day, which means they fast for the recommended 16 hours.

Of course, it isn't as bad as it sounds since they are sleeping during this time, so what it comes down to is eating dinner and then not eating the next day again around lunch, so you are just skipping breakfast.

You will be doing it every day, so finding the hours that work for you are important. If you work the third shift, then switching you're eating period around to fit into your schedule is important. If you find yourself being run down and sluggish, tweak your fasting hours until you find a healthy balance. Granted, there will be some adjustment because chances are, your body is not accustomed to skipping entire meals. However, this should go away after a couple of weeks, and if it doesn't, then try starting your fasting period earlier in the day, allowing you to eat earlier the next, or alter it however you need to feel healthy and happy.

LEAN-GAINS METHOD (14:10)

The lean-gains method has several different incarnations on the web, but its fame comes from the fact that it helps shed fat while building it into muscle almost immediately. Through the lean-gains method, you'll find yourself able to shift all that fat to be muscle through a rigorous practice of fasting, eating right, and exercising.

Through this method, you fast anywhere from 14 to 16 hours and spend the remaining 10 or 8 hours each day engaged in eating and exercise. As opposed to the crescendo, this method features daily fasting and eating, rather than alternated days of eating versus not. Therefore, you don't have to be quite cautious about extending the physical effort to exercise on the days you are fasting because those days when you're fasting are every day!

For the lean-gaining method, start fasting only for 14 hours and work it up to 16 if you feel comfortable with it, but never forget to drink enough water and be careful about spending too much energy on exercise! Remember that you want to grow in health and potential through intermittent fasting. You'll certainly not want to lose any of that growth by forcing the process along.

20:4 METHOD

Stepping things up a notch from the 14:10 and 16:8 methods, the 20:4 method is a tough one to master, for it is rather unforgiving. People talk about this method of intermittent fasting as intense and highly restrictive. Still, they also say that the effects of living this method are almost unparalleled with all other tactics.

For the 20:4 method, you'll fast for 20 hours each day and squeeze all your meals, all your eating, and all your snacking into 4 hours. People who attempt 20:4 normally have two smaller meals or just one large meal and a few snacks during their 4-hour window to eat, and it is up to the individual which four hours of the day they devote to eating.

The trick for this method is to make sure you're not overeating or bingeing during those 4-hour windows to eat. It is all-too-easy to get hungry during the 20-hour fast and have that feeling then propel you into intense and unrealistic hunger or meal sizes after the fast period is over. Be careful if you try this method. If you're new to intermittent fasting, work your way up to this one gradually, and if you're working your way up already, only make the shift to 20:4 when you know you're ready. It would surely disappoint if all your progress with intermittent fasting got hijacked by one poorly thought-out goal with the 20:4 method.

MEAL SKIPPING

Meal skipping is an extremely flexible form of intermittent fasting that can provide all of the benefits of intermittent fasting but with less strict scheduling. If you are not someone who has a typical schedule or feels like a stricter variation of the intermittent fasting diet will serve you, meal skipping is a viable alternative.

Many people who choose to use meal skipping find it a great way to listen to their bodies and follow their basic instincts. If they are not hungry, they simply don't eat that meal. Instead, they wait for the next one. Meal skipping can also help people who have time constraints and who may not always be able to get in a certain meal of the day.

It is important to realize that with meal skipping, you may not always be maintaining a 10-16-hour window of fasting. As a result, you may not get every benefit that comes from other fasting diets. However, this may be a great solution for people who want an intermittent fasting diet that feels more natural. It may also be a great idea for those looking to begin listening to their bodies more so that they can adjust to a more extreme variant of the diet with greater ease. It can be a great transitional diet for you if you are not ready to jump into one of the other fasting diets just yet.

WARRIOR DIET FASTING

The most extreme form of intermittent fasting is known as the Warrior Diet. This intermittent fasting cycle follows a 20-hour fasting window with a short 4-hour eating window. During that eating window, individuals are supposed only to consume raw fruits and vegetables. They can also eat one large meal. Typically, the eating window occurs at night time, so people can snack throughout the evening, have a large meal, and then resume fasting.

Because of the length of fasting taking place during the Warrior Diet, people should also consume a fairly hearty level of healthy fats. Doing so will give the body something to consume during the fast to produce energy with. Additional carbohydrates are also used to increase energy levels; too.

People who eat the Warrior Diet tend to believe that humans are natural nocturnal eaters and that we are not meant to eat throughout the day. The belief is that eating this way follows our natural circadian rhythms, allowing our body to work optimally.

The only people who should consider doing the Warrior Diet are those who have already had success with other forms of intermittent fasting and who are used to it. Attempting to jump straight into the Warrior Diet can have serious repercussions for anyone who is not used to intermittent fasting. Even still, those who are used to it may find this particular style too extreme for them to maintain.

EAT-STOP-EAT (24 HOUR) METHOD

This method of fasting is incredibly similar to the crescendo method. The only discernable difference is that there's no anticipation of increasing into a more intense fasting pattern with time. For the eat-stop-eat method, you decide which days you want to take off from eating, and then you run with it until you've lost that weight, and then you keep running with the lifestyle for good because you won't be able to imagine life without it.

The eat-stop-eat method involves one to two days a week being 100% oriented towards fasting, with the other five to six days concerning "business as normal." The one or two days spent fasting are then full 24-hour days spent without eating anything at all. These days, of course, water and coffee are still fine to drink, but no food items can be consumed whatsoever. Exercise is also frowned upon on those fasting days but see what your body can handle before you decide how that should all work out.

Some people might start thinking they're using the crescendo method but end up sticking with eat-stop-eat.

ALTERNATE-DAY METHOD

The alternate-day method is admittedly a little confusing, but the reason it could be so confusing could come, in part, from how much wiggle room it provides for the practitioner. This method is great for people who don't have a consistent schedule or any sense of one; it is incredibly forgiving for those who don't quite have everything together for themselves yet.

When it comes down to it, alternate-day intermittent fasting is really up to you. You should try to fast every other day, but it doesn't have to be that precise. Similarly, with the crescendo method, as long as you fast two to three days a week, with a break day or two in between each fasting day, you're set! Then, you'll want to eat normally for three or four days out of each week, and when you encounter a fasting day, you don't even need to completely fast!

Alternate-day fasting is a solid place to start from, especially if you work a varying schedule or still have yet to get used to a consistent one. If you want to make things more intense from this starting point, the alternate-day method can easily become the eat-stop-eat method, the crescendo method, or the 5:2 method. Essentially, this method is a great place to begin

12:12 METHOD

As another of the more natural ways of intermittent fasting, the 12:12 approach is well-suited to beginning practitioners. Many people live out the 12:12 method without any forethought simply because of their sleeping and eating schedule, but turning 12:12 into a conscious practice can have just as many positive effects on your life as the more drastic 20:4 method claims.

According to a study conducted in the University of Alabama, for this method, in particular, you fast for 12 hours and then enter a 12-hour eating window. It's not difficult whatsoever to get three small meals and several snacks, or two big meals and a snack into your day with this method. With 12:12, the standard meal timing works just fine.

Ultimately, this method is a great one to start from, for a lot of variation can be built into this scheduling when you're ready to make things more interesting. Effortlessly and without much effort, 12:12 can become 14:10 or even 16:8, and in seemingly no time, you can find yourself trying alternate-day or crescendo methods, too. Start with what's normal for you, and this method might be exactly that!

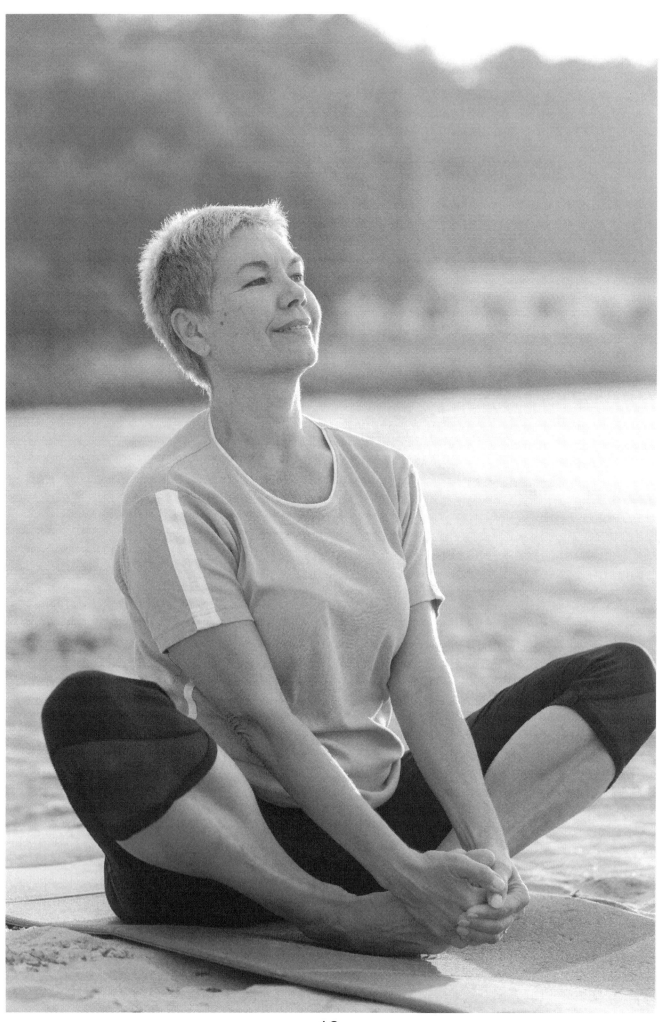

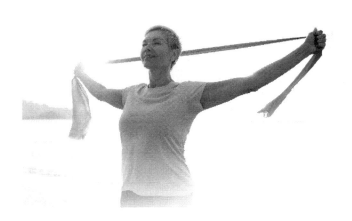

HEALTH BENEFITS OF INTERMITTENT FASTING

When women get to 50 and over, their skin will start to show signs of age. They may find their joints start to ache for no reason, and suddenly belly fat accumulates as if you have just given birth. There are so many creams, diets and exercises on the market to tighten the skin and try to help. The fact is, they may work to a certain point but then the body hits a shelf, and nothing seems to push a person past it.

This boils up frustration making women look into the more drastic and very expensive alternatives like surgery.

Which in itself poses so many more dangers and risks for women of 50 and over.

A person does not need to go under the knife or starve themselves to reboot their system or change their shape. Intermittent fasting is a much cheaper and less risky way to do this and there is no need to make any drastic eating habits changes either. Well, you may need to make a few adjustments like cutting out junk food and eating healthier. But once again the diet a person follows is their personal choice and depends on how serious they are about becoming healthier.

Some health benefits of intermittent fasting for women over 50 include:

ACTIVATING CELLULAR REPAIR

Fasting has been known to kick start the body's natural cellular repair function, get rid of mature cells, improve longevity, and improve hormone function. All things that tend to take a battering as people age. This can alleviate joint and muscle aches as well as lower back pain. As the cells are being repaired and the damage is undone, it helps with the skin's elasticity and health too.

Increase Cognitive Function and Protects the Brain from Damage

Intermittent fasting may increase the levels of a brain hormone known as a brain-derived neurotrophic factor (BDNF). It may equally guard the brain against damage like a stroke or Alzheimer's disease as it promotes new nerve cell growth. It also increases cognitive function and could effectively defend a person against other neurodegenerative diseases as well.

WEIGHT LOSS

When people have belly fat, it can cause many health problems that are associated with various diseases as it indicates a person has visceral fat. Visceral fat is fat that goes deep into the abdominal surrounding the organs. Belly fat is terribly hard to lose, especially for an aging woman. Intermittent fasting has been known to help reduce not only weight but inches of over five percent of body fat in around twenty-two to twenty-five weeks (Barna, 2019).

ALLEVIATES OXIDATIVE STRESS AND INFLAMMATION

Oxidative stress is when the body has an imbalance of antioxidants as well as free radicals. This imbalance can cause both tissue and cell damage in overweight as well as aging people. It can also lead to various chronic illnesses like cancer, heart disease, diabetes, and also has an impact on the signs of aging. Oxidative stress can trigger the inflammation that causes these diseases.

Intermittent fasting can provide your system with a reboot, helping to alleviate oxidative stress and inflammation in a middle-aged woman. It also significantly reduces the risk of oxidative stress and inflammation for those overweight or obese.

SLOW DOWN THE AGING PROCESS

As intermittent fasting gives both the metabolism and cellular repair a reboot it offers the potential to slow down aging. It may even prolong a person's lifespan by quite a few years especially if following a nutritious diet and exercise regime alongside intermittent fasting.

ULTIMATE STEPS FOR GETTING STARTED

Although intermittent fasting is a very simple and straightforward approach yet, fasting can be an intimidating word for many. Our dependence on food for our physical, mental, and emotional satisfaction has increased to such an extent that even the thought of abstinence from food can make people anxious. This is even more important in the case of women as controlling hunger for them can be very difficult. Their mind is internally programmed to look for food consciously.

This is a reason that although intermittent fasting is very easy and simple, some people may find it difficult to follow it in the long run.

The main reason some people may find intermittent fasting difficult to follow is not due to the severity of hunger or their inability to manage their routine but because they have not followed proper procedures.

Yes, you have read it right! The biggest reason people are unable to follow intermittent fasting is that they don't follow the process properly. They are so enthusiastic about losing weight that they don't give time to their bodies to prepare for the fasting schedules.

You must understand that humans have also evolved from animal species. Our first and foremost instinct is and always would be to eat, sleep, and procreate. If any hindrance is put in the way of either of these things, the initial reaction of our body would be adverse. If you try to snatch away any of these things or enforce stricter rules in these areas, the results are not going to be favorable.

No matter how beneficial fasting is for the body, the body is not going to react well to it initially. You will face the hunger pangs, cramps, distraction, mind wandering around food, irritability, and mood swings. There are ways to manage all these symptoms, but there can be no denying the fact that these issues will arise.

You can lower these adverse reactions by following proper protocols, and intermittent fasting will become a life-changing experience for you. If you jump the steps and rush to the last part in the first leg, you are bound to have severe symptoms, and not only the results would get affected, but you will also face problems in managing the lifestyle for long.

A STEP-BY-STEP APPROACH

The best way to approach intermittent fasting is to move step by step. You must never undermine the fact that our lifestyles are heavily centered on food. There are shorter gaps between meals. There is a high amount of carb-intake that also aggravates the situation to a great extent.

If you follow a very hard approach from the word GO, you are bound to face adjustment issues. The best approach is to allow the body to adapt to the fasting schedule and let it build the capacity to stay hungry.

Eliminate Snacks

This is something that would come several times in this book. It is a very important thing that you must understand. The root cause of most of our health issues is the habit of frequent snacking.

Snacking leads to 2 major issues:

1. It keeps causing repeated glucose spikes that invoke an insulin response and hence the overall insulin presence in the bloodstream increases aggravating the problem of insulin resistance.

2. It usually involves refined carb and sugar-rich food items that will lead to cravings and you will keep feeling the urge to eat at even shorter intervals.

This is a reason your preparation for intermittent fasting must begin with the elimination of snacks. You can have 2-3 nutrient-dense meals in a day, but you will have to remove the habit of snacking from your routine.

As long as the habit of snacking is there, you'll have a very hard time staying away from food as this habit never allows your ghrelin response clock to get set at fixed intervals. This means that you will keep having urges to eat sweets and carb-rich foods, and you will also have strong hunger pangs at regular intervals.

The solution to this problem is very simple. You can take 2-3 nutrient-dense meals that are rich in fat, protein, and fiber. Such a meal will not only provide you with adequate energy for the day but would also keep your gut engaged for long so that you don't have frequent hunger pangs.

The farther you can stay away from refined carb-rich and sugar-rich food items, the easier you would find it to deal with hunger.

You must start easy. Don't do anything drastic or earth-shattering.

Simply start by lowering the number of snacks you have in a day. The snacks have not only become a need of the body, but they are also a part of the habit. In a day, there are numerous instances when we eat tit-bits that we don't care about. We sip cold-drinks, sweetened beverages, chips, cookies, bagels, donuts, burgers, pizzas simply because they are in front of us or accessible. We have made food an excuse to take breaks. This habit will have to be broken if you want to move on the path of good health.

Widen the Gap between Your Meals

This is the second step in your preparation. You must start widening the gap between your meals. This process needs to be gradual and should only begin when you have eliminated snacks from your routine. Two nutrient-dense meals in a day or two meals and a smaller meal or lunch comprising of fiber-rich salads should be your goal.

However, you must remember that these two steps must be taken over a long period. You must allow your body to get used to the change. There would be a temptation that it is easy to follow these, and you can jump to the actual intermittent fasting routine, but it is very important to avoid all such temptations as they are only going to lead to failures.

If your body doesn't get used to this routine, very soon, you'll start feeling trapped. You'll start finding ways to cheat the routine. You'll look for excuses to violate the routine, and it very soon becomes a habit. This is the reason you must allow your body to take some time to adjust to the new schedule.

You should remember that intermittent fasting is a way of life. This might slower the results, but it is going to make your overall journey smoother and better.

INSIDER TIPS FOR BREAKING A FAST

How you break, your fast will depend on the time of day at which it occurs and the type of fast that you participated in. Here, I will go over some general rules fort breaking your fast, but keep in mind that you will need to adjust these slightly to fit your personal fast. The important things to keep in mind are the same among all fasts, however.

Breaking your fast is all about showing your body that you are not undergoing starvation and that there is not going to be an ongoing lack of food, but that it is going to have to become used to eating less often than it used to. After some time, it will adjust to this, but in the beginning, it will be attempting to keep you alive as it thinks that there has been some type of food drought.

There are specific times when it is most important to break your fast in a very deliberate way.

These times are closer to the beginning of your introduction of fasting, when you change the duration of fasting if you are working your way up to longer fasts and when you fast for the first time in a while.

While it is always important to break your fast with clear guidelines, at these times, it is most important as the chances of experiencing some stomach upset post-fast are the highest. Follow the guidelines below to see what things you should be keeping in mind when you break your fast.

Start with Water

If you are breaking fast in the morning, begin by drinking a glass of water before anything else. This will put something into your stomach and tell your body that it is time to begin working for the day. If you are breaking fast in the evening and have been drinking water all day, stick to water with your meal as you don't want to feed your digestive system too much at once.

Break Fast Slowly

While eating your first meal, you will likely feel the urge to eat very quickly and eat as much as you can, as faster as you can, as it has been a while since you last ate. It is important to control this urge as you may experience some bloating or discomfort in the digestion of your food.

Practice mindfulness while eating. This means taking every bite slowly and ensuring that you taste and chew each bite fully. Take note of how the food feels in your mouth and how it tastes. Remain in the present moment, focused on the bite you are taking, and try not to think of anything else. Since you have not eaten in a while, try to enjoy the first meal you have after you fast. Instead of eating it so quickly that you don't even remember the taste of it, take your time to savor it.

THINGS TO WATCH OUT FOR

If you make the decision that fasting is right for you, there may be a time during your fast that you must seek medical advice. Knowing when to seek medical advice and when you may be dealing with regular side-effects of fasting is important to ensure you are fasting in a healthy manner.

Side-effects that signal for you to consult a doctor

- Nausea
- Dizziness
- Bloody stools
- Vomiting
- Loss of consciousness
- Abdominal or chest pain

If any of the above symptoms happens to you while fasting, consult a doctor as there may be some complications or other problems that fasting has brought about.

If you experience diarrhea, this may be caused by a number of things, but more importantly, diarrhea can lead to other more serious issues like dehydration, dizziness, cramping, and malnutrition. If you experience diarrhea while fasting, you can end your fast and see if this clears up though home methods such as hydrating, restoring electrolytes, and consuming potassium-rich foods. If it does, consider trying another kind of fast or visiting your doctor to determine other, safer ways to fast. However, if you are experiencing severe diarrhea, along with any pains or severe dehydration, contact a doctor immediately.

COMMON MISTAKES TO AVOID

Making Lots of Changes within a Short Duration

It is natural to get too excited when you are about to start something new; you can't wait to have all the rewards that come with it, so you probably want to dive into it. However, you need to caution that trying to make lots of changes in a few weeks can prevent you from enjoying all the rewards you seek. Hence, you must start slowly and grow into it; an instance is adopting the 5:2 method where you eat only 500 calories all through the day twice in a week and feed "normal" on the remaining five days. You may start by eating 500 calories once in the week and having regular meals for the remaining six days. After 2-3 weeks, you can add the second day, and from there, you can adopt other methods with more extended fasting periods.

Not Monitoring Your Liquid Intake

It is essential to know that your fasting state can come to an end not only when you eat, but also when you drink the liquids, you are not supposed to. Some liquids will break your fast and deny you the fast benefits, even if they are calorie or fat-free. Diet sodas and sweeteners are some of the liquids you should stay away from; sweetener can cause a spike in your insulin levels.

The main liquid you are permitted to take while doing intermittent fasting is water. Moderate black coffee is also allowed. Adding lemon to your water or sugar to the coffee will also nullify your fast.

Not Drinking Adequate Water

It is recommended to drink a lot of water while engaging in intermittent fasting. If you refuse to drink enough water while fasting, it can make you dehydrated and very thirsty, and it is possible to confuse thirst for hunger. The International Food Information has already stated that 20% of the water the body uses comes from the foods we feed on. At the same time, since you are intermittent fasting, your food intake will be limited; hence, you need to drink 20% more water than usual to make up for the foods.

Feeding on Unhealthy Foods

Intermittent fasting is not a diet plan; hence, it doesn't prevent you from eating your food choice. The freedom of having the luxury to eat any meal has made a lot of people fall into a "trap" as they feed on junks or breaking their fast with fast food. Desist from the habit of feeding on unhealthy meals with the mindset that your fasts would cover up for you.

To enjoy all the health benefits of intermittent fasting, it is essential to feed on healthy foods. When you visit the grocery store, buy foods rich in protein, calcium, and B-12.

Overeating When You Break Your Fast

This is a prevalent mistake most beginners of intermittent fasting make. Even those who practice intermittent fasting in the past and claim it doesn't work mostly do this. If you eat lots of calorie-filled meals when you break your fast and are trying to lose weight, you probably might not be able to achieve your aim.

To avoid overeating, you should feed on large quantities of healthy foods during your eating period. This food should be made up of fresh vegetables and healthy salads. You should also have your meal prepared before your fasting period ends; this will prevent you from eating just anything when your fasting period elapsed.

Sticking with the Wrong Plan

There are several plans for intermittent fasting. It is essential to study each of these plans and adopt one that can easily be integrated into your daily routine. If your work requires you to leave home very early in the morning to engage in strenuous jobs, the fasting plan whereby you won't eat from 8 pm until after 12 pm the following day will be a wrong plan for you as this will not augur well with your job.

It is essential to know that the intermittent fasting plan that works for someone else might not work for you. Hence, you can experiment with the various methods available and study each of them as it applies to you to see the one that gives you the best result.

PROVEN TIPS FOR MANAGING YOUR FAST

Each segment will cover the practical tips that are needed to manage your days of fasting. If you continue with your intermittent fasting regime, these will benefit you.

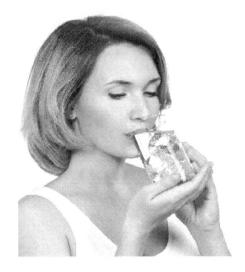

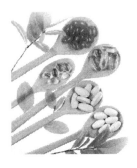

*1.***When you get hungry**, hunger suppressants help you get through the fasting window when you get thirsty. These include coffee, sugar, green tea, cinnamon and chia seeds. Use these in order to help you get through!

*3.***Getting tired or dizzy:** This is usually due to dehydration, so make sure you're drinking plenty. Increasing your salt intake is also advisable–particularly if headaches become a concern.

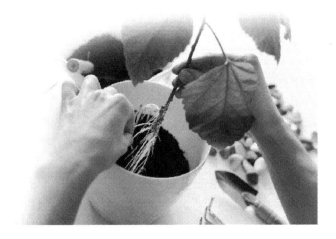

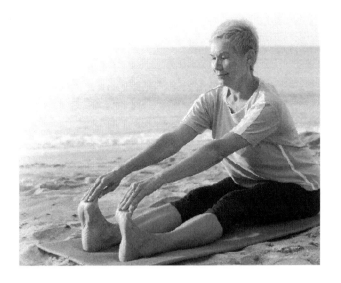

*2.***The mixture of diet and exercise:** This is possible; several tests have shown that it's okay! You're going to work out what time of day is better for your training after a while

*4.***I'm struggling here:** The best way to avoid giving up is to stay busy. By getting out and doing something constructive, take your mind off food.

*5.***I'm too busy:** This can be for your benefit because your focus is not always going to be on food. Prepare a quick that matches the current hours of work / commitments before this becomes troublesome. There's no reason for not doing that–particularly not that.

6. **I'm going to gorge:** Once you've accomplished your fast, assume that it never happened and continue as normal. When time goes by, this will make it easier and the body will be adapted.

7. **Things continue to crop up**: That's why it's essential to prepare. Clearing your calendar with crucial things and adapting will be the same as how effective you are.

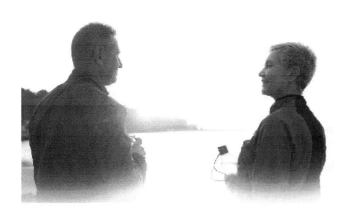

8. **Meeting with the negativity:** Not everyone knows the effects of fasting, so it's best to educate those who need to hear about it–relatives, close friends, etc. Others are going to try to put you off or freak you out, stopping you from setting off.

9. **Maintaining the loss of weight:** The fast is not a quick fix. It's a long-term change in lifestyle that will help you keep the slimmer/healthier image you love. It's also best to eat much better and keep this up all the way.

How to keep going: You need to relax if you feel tired. There's something the body is trying to tell you and you need to listen. That's why it's recommended that you clear your schedule at the outset.

FREQUENTLY ASKED QUESTIONS ABOUT INTERMITTENT FASTING

IS INTERMITTENT FASTING DIFFICULT TO ADHERE TO?

It could be difficult for some people. You may experience difficulties and challenges especially if you are still a beginner and your body still adjust and adapts to the new routine and pattern of food intake. Once your body adapts, you will find the eating pattern more manageable and easier to follow.

The main premise is being more aware of when and what you should eat. With such awareness, you will know exactly the boundaries and limitations you have to keep in mind. Also, it would be best to pair this approach with daily exercise and making healthy food choices, like fruits, beans, veggies, healthy fats, lean proteins, and lentils.

Avoiding too much sugar and sodium is a must, too. Once your body adapts to these new guidelines, adhering to IF will no longer be that challenging.

WHAT IS THE RECOMMENDED NUMBER OF HOURS/DAYS FOR FASTING?

In most cases, followers of the IF approach set their fasting window to up to 16 hours daily. Most follow this routine as it is a bit easy to adapt and adhere to. You can do it just by skipping breakfast after you ate your last meal the other day. If you can, you may also practice the IF pattern, which requires you to go without food for 24 hours straight twice every week.

DO I STILL NEED TO COUNT CALORIES?

The answer to this will depend on the goals you want to achieve while practicing IF. It is not necessary in some cases but if your goal is to lose weight, then you may want to monitor your calorie intake still.

Also, if you plan to cut out on snacks before sleeping or go without eating for a long period, then you will notice your calorie count declining naturally. Another thing to note is that taking in foods that are mostly plant-based will also naturally lower your calorie intake.

SHOULD WOMEN DO IF DIFFERENTLY?

In most cases, men and women tend to respond differently to the IF protocol. Most women also agree that they tend to achieve better results by widening their eating window a bit. For instance, when trying to follow the 16/8 IF plan, some women noticed that they get better results after they modified the approach – that is increasing the number of eating hours to 10 and reducing the fasting hours to 14.

A wise advice is to experiment and find out which one works for you. Observe the signals and cues sent by your body. Determine how it reacts to a specific IF pattern, too. Make sure to stick to an approach that seems to stimulate positive and favorable responses from your body.

IS IT SAFE FOR PREGNANT OR BREASTFEEDING WOMEN TO FAST?

Intermittent fasting is not highly recommended for pregnant women. It is mainly because your focus during pregnancy should be to supply your body with nutrients that can support your health and the growth and development of your baby. You need to eat highly nutritious foods that will help develop and build your baby's body and brains.

Also, take note that there are pregnant women who have a hard time having enough iron stores. If you do not eat the required foods every day, then it might lead to iron deficiency, which is important for your baby. Despite that, there is still no rule that bans pregnant women from practicing IF.

If you are one of those who have already practiced it and your health is at its best, then following IF is most likely safe for you. Just make sure that you only do it after receiving the consent from your doctor. Also, it would be best to shorten the fasting period. If you are used to doing it for 24 hours or more, then avoid doing it while you are pregnant. You should fast for at most 14 to 16 hours only.

If you are breastfeeding, long fasting periods also need to be avoided. It is because of the constant need of your baby for nutritional milk. Fasting may have a huge impact on the quality and production of breast milk so you have to be extra careful. A wise advice is to avoid fasting for more than 12 to 14 hours if you are breastfeeding to ensure that the production of milk will not be interrupted.

Make sure to observe yourself and the body, too. If you notice that your milk supply suddenly dries up and you suspect that it is because of IF, then stop fasting right away. Try to eat more regularly to find out if doing so resolves the issue. If you notice fasting greatly hampering your milk production, then maybe it is time to stop it for a while and just continue once you already stop breastfeeding.

CAN I STILL WORK OUT EVEN IF I AM DOING IF?

Of course, you can. If your fasting period is 24 hours or more, then you may want to schedule your workouts during your non-fasting days to ensure that you have more energy to complete the sessions. You can also see other women working out even during their fasting periods, especially if their fasting takes less than 24 hours.

It is because they notice how effective exercising during a fast is in building lean muscle mass. In general, you should schedule your exercise based on how your body feels as well as the workout habits you are used to.

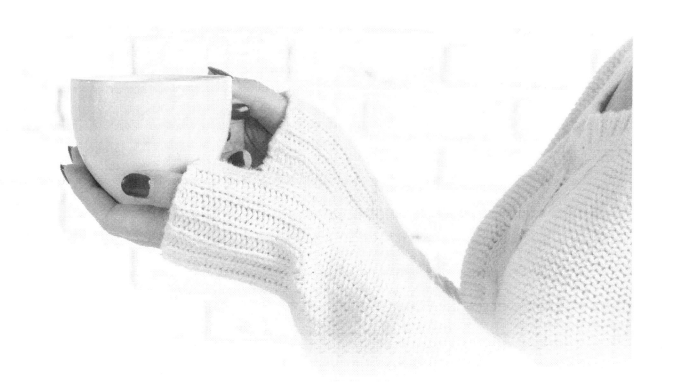

BREAKFAST FOR YOUR INTERMITTENT FAST

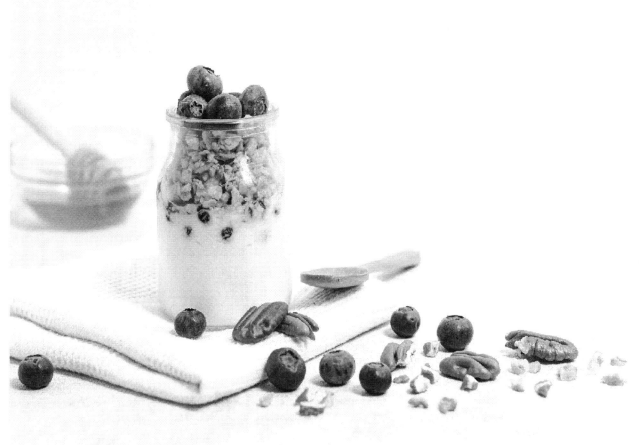

Healthy Chia and Oats Smoothie

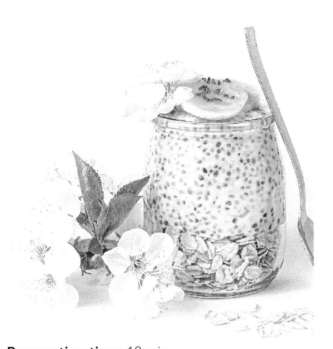

Preparation time: 10 min

Cooking time: 0 minutes

Servings: 2

Nutrition:

- calories 140,
- fat 7,
- fiber 4,
- carbs 12,
- protein 12

Ingredients:

6 tbsp. oats

2 tbsp. chia seeds

2 tbsp. hemp powder

4 medjool dates, pitted (optional)

2 bananas, chopped

1 cup almond milk

Direction

1. Add all the ingredients in a blender and blend until smooth.
2. Pour in glasses and serve.

Cherry Almond and Cereal Smoothie

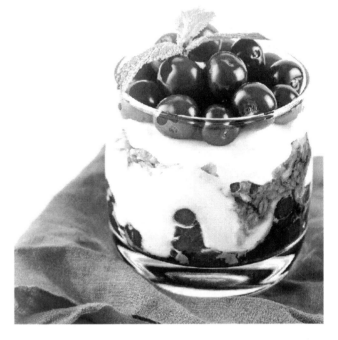

Preparation time: 10 min

Cooking time: 0 minutes

Servings: 2

Nutrition:

- calories 200,
- fat 8g,
- fiber 4g,
- carbs 8g,
- protein 3g

Ingredients:

1 cup fresh cherries, pitted + extra to garnish

¼ cup rolled oats

1 tbsp. hemp seeds

1 cup almond milk

Direction:

1. Add all the ingredients in a blender and blend until smooth.
2. Pour into glasses and serve garnished with cherries.

Banana Orange Smoothie

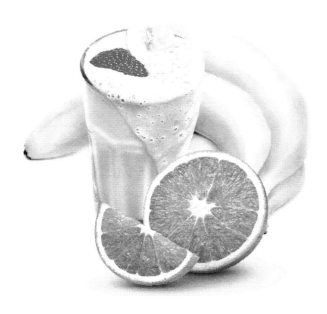

Preparation time: 10 minutes

Cooking time: 0 minutes

Servings: 2

Nutrition:
- calories 183,
- fat 8g,
- fiber 1g,
- carbs 3g,
- protein 9g

Ingredients:

2 cups fat free milk

1 cup nonfat Greek yogurt

1 medium banana

1 cup collard greens

1 orange, peeled, deseeded, separated into segments

6 strawberries, chopped

2 tbsp. sesame seeds

Direction:

1. Add all the ingredients in a blender and blend until smooth.
2. Pour in glasses and serve.

Crunchy Banana Yoghurt

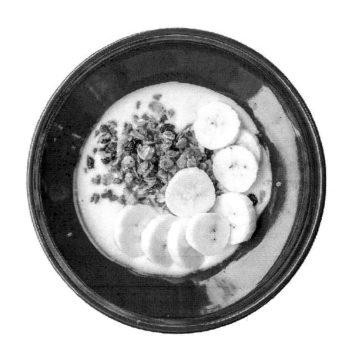

Preparation time: 10 min

Cooking time: 0 minutes

Servings: 4

Nutrition:
- calories 323,
- fat 11g,
- fiber 4g,
- carbs 13g,
- protein 17g

Ingredients:

3 cups fat free natural Greek style yogurt

1 ounce mixed seeds or nuts of your choice like pumpkin seeds etc.

2 bananas, sliced

Direction:

1. Take 4 bowls and add ¾ cup yogurt into each bowl.
2. Divide the banana slices among the bowl.
3. Sprinkle seeds on top and serve.

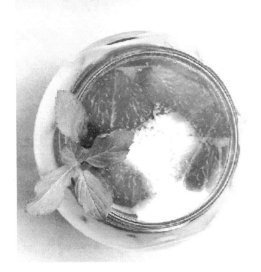

Grapefruit Yogurt Parfait

Preparation time: 10 min

Cooking time: 5 minutes

Servings: 4

Nutrition:
- calories 103g,
- fat 4g,
- fiber 1g,
- carbs 3g,
- protein 22g

Ingredients:

½ cup amaranth

1 grapefruit, peeled, separated into segments, deseeded, chopped

3 tbsp. toasted coconut

Stevia to taste (optional)

1 cup plain, nonfat yogurt

Direction:

1. Place a pan over medium heat. Add amaranth and let it pop. It should take 3-5 minutes. Let it cool for a few minutes.
2. Add yogurt into a bowl. Add stevia and stir. Add 2 tbsp. yogurt into each of 4 glasses.
3. Place a layer of grapefruit in each glass. Add 1 tbsp. popped amaranth and sprinkle some coconut into the glasses.
4. Repeat steps 2-3 until all the ingredients are used up.

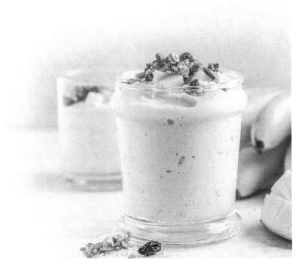

Creamy Mango and Banana Overnight Oats

Preparation time: 10 minutes

Cooking time: 0 minutes

Servings: 1

Nutrition:
- calories 199,
- fat 8g,
- fiber 4g,
- carbs 9g,
- protein 4g

Ingredients:

For the smoothie:

1 ripe banana

½ mango, peeled, cubed

½ tbsp. ground flaxseed

1 cup almond milk

For the oats:

1/3 cup oats

1 small ripe banana, mashed

1/2 cup almond milk

½ tbsp. ground flaxseed

2 tbsp. chia seeds

Stevia or erythritol to taste

Direction:

1. Add all the smoothie ingredients into a blender and blend until smooth.
2. Pour into a tall glass.
3. To make the oats layer: Add oats, almond milk, flaxseed, chia seeds and stevia into a bowl. Stir well and add banana. Mix until well combined. Pour it over the smoothie in the glass.
4. Chill in the refrigerator overnight and serve.

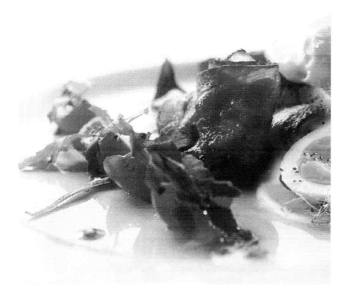

BACON AND EGGS WITH TOMATOES

Preparation time: 10 min
Cooking time: 30 minutes
Servings: 5

Nutrition:
- calories 110,
- fat 10g,
- fiber 1g,
- carbs 3g,
- protein 6g

Ingredients:

4 large ripe tomatoes, halved
8 rashers smoked back bacon, trimmed of fat
4 eggs
Salt to taste
Pepper to taste
1 tsp. vinegar

Direction:

1. Set up the grill to preheat. Let it preheat to high heat.
2. Place a rack on the grill pan. Line the pan with foil. Place tomatoes on the rack. Let it grill for 3 minutes. Place bacon along with the tomatoes.
3. Grill for 4 minutes until soft.
4. Meanwhile, place a large saucepan over medium high heat. Fill the saucepan up to about ¾ with water. Let it boil.
5. When it begins to boil, add vinegar and stir. Crack an egg into a bowl and slowly slide the egg into the boiling water. Repeat this, one at a time.
6. Cook each egg until it is soft boiled, for 2-3 minutes.
7. Meanwhile, divide the bacon and tomatoes into 2 plates.
8. Remove the eggs with a slotted spoon and place on the plates. Sprinkle salt and pepper and serve.

CINNAMON PORRIDGE

Preparation time: 10 min
Cooking time: 30 min
Servings: 4

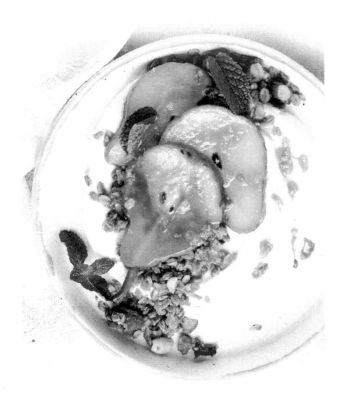

Cinnamon and Pecan Porridge

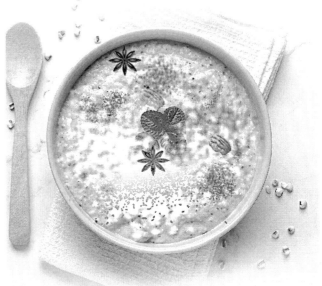

Preparation time: 5 minutes

Cooking time: 10 minutes

Servings: 2

Nutrition:
- calories 580,
- fat 14g,
- fiber 10g,
- carbs 3g,
- protein 8g

Nutrition:
- calories 383,
- fat 14g,
- fiber 4g,
- carbs 3g,
- protein 8g

Ingredients:

4 ½ ounces jumbo porridge oats

20 ounces semi-skimmed milk

1 tsp. lemon juice

½ tsp. ground cinnamon + extra to garnish

2 ripe medium pears, peeled, cored, grated

Direction:

1. Add oats, milk and cinnamon into a nonstick saucepan. Place the saucepan over medium low heat. Cook until creamy. Stir constantly.
2. Divide into bowls. Scatter pear on top. Drizzle lemon juice on top. Garnish with cinnamon and serve.

Ingredients

½ tsp. cinnamon

¼ cup pecans, chopped

¼ cup unsweetened coconut, toasted

¼ cup coconut milk

¼ cup almond butter

¾ cup unsweetened almond milk

1 tbsp. extra virgin coconut oil

2 tbsps. Hemp seeds

2 tbsps. Whole chia seeds

Directions

1. Place a small saucepan over medium heat. Combine the coconut milk, coconut oil, almond butter, and almond milk. Bring to simmer and remove from heat.

2. Add the toasted coconut (leave some for the topping), cinnamon, pecans, hemp seeds, and chia seeds. Mix the ingredients well and allow to rest for 5-10 minutes.

3. Divide between two bowls and serve.

FETA-FILLED TOMATO-TOPPED OLDIE OMELET

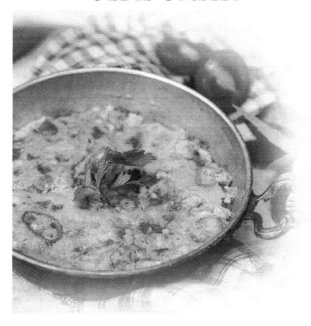

Preparation Time: 5 minutes
Cooking Time: 6 minutes
Servings: 1

Nutrition:
- Calories: 335,
- Fat: 28.4 g
- Protein: 16.2 g
- Carbs: 4.5 g
- Fiber: 0.8 g

Ingredients:
1 tablespoon coconut oil
2 pcs eggs
1½ tablespoon milk
A dash of salt and pepper
¼ cup tomatoes, sliced into cubes
2 tablespoons feta cheese, crumbled

Directions:
1. Beat the eggs with the pepper, salt, milk, and the remaining spices.
2. Pour the mixture into a heated pan with coconut oil.
3. Stir in the tomatoes and cheese. Cook for 6 minutes or until the cheese melts.

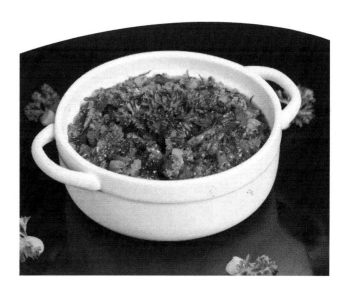

CARROT BREAKFAST SALAD

Preparation Time: 5 minutes
Cooking Time: 4 hours
Servings: 4

Nutrition:
- Calories: 437,
- Protein: 2.39 grams,
- Fat: 39.14 grams
- Carbs: 23.28 grams

Ingredients:

- 2 tablespoons olive oil
- 2 pounds' baby carrots, peeled and halved
- 3 garlic cloves, minced
- 3 celery stalks, chopped
- 2 yellow onions, chopped
- ½ cup vegetable stock
- 1/3 cup tomatoes, crushed
- A pinch of salt and black pepper

Directions:

1. In your slow cooker, combine all the ingredients, cover and cook on high for 4 hours.
2. Divide into bowls and serve for breakfast.

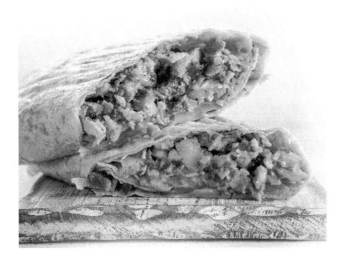

Delicious Turkey Wrap

Preparation Time: 10 minutes
Cooking Time: 10 minutes
Servings: 6

Nutrition:

- Calories: 162,
- Fat: 4 g
- Carbohydrates: 7 g
- Protein: 23 g

Ingredients:

1 and a ¼ pounds of ground turkey, lean

4 green onions, minced
1 tablespoon of olive oil
1 garlic clove, minced
2 teaspoons of chili paste
8 ounces water chestnut, diced
3 tablespoons of hoisin sauce
2 tablespoons of coconut amino
1 tablespoon of rice vinegar
12 butter lettuce leaves
1/8 teaspoon of salt

Directions:

1. Take a pan and place it over medium heat, add turkey and garlic to the pan
2. Heat for 6 minutes until cooked
3. Take a bowl and transfer turkey to the bowl
4. Add onions and water chestnuts
5. Stir in hoisin sauce, coconut amino, vinegar, and chili paste
6. Toss well and transfer the mix to lettuce leaves. Serve and enjoy.

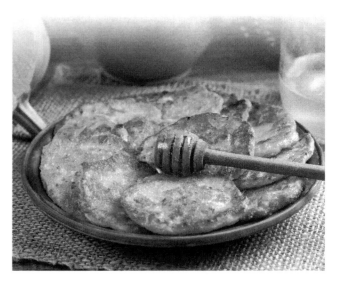

Pumpkin Pancakes

Preparation Time: 10 min
Cooking Time: 15 min
Servings: 6

Nutrition:
- Calories: 70,
- Carbs: 16 g
- Fat: 3 g
- Protein: 3 g

Ingredients:

3 Large eggs - Separate the egg whites for use

2/3 cups of organic oats

6 ounces' pumpkin puree

1 scoop of collagen peptides

1 teaspoon stevia powder

½ teaspoon cinnamon

Cooking spray

Directions:

1. Blend all the ingredients into a smooth mixture.
2. Apply the cooking spray to the pan to coat it properly.
3. Pour a part of the batter into the pan and let it coat the pan properly
4. Wait till the edges of the pancake brown up a little bit
5. Flip it over and cook from the other side

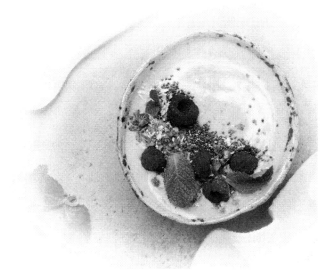

CHERRY SMOOTHIE BOWL

Preparation Time: 15 minutes

Cooking Time: 0 minute

Servings: 1

Nutrition:

Calories: 130,

Carbs: 32 g

Fat: 5g

Protein: 1 g

Ingredients:

(Soak the organic rolled oats in half a cup of unsweetened almond milk)

- ½ cup of organic rolled oats
- ½ cup almond milk-unsweetened
- 1 tablespoon Chia seeds
- 2 teaspoons granola
- 2 teaspoons almonds sliced
- 1 tablespoon almond butter
- 1 teaspoon vanilla extract
- ½ cup berries-fresh
- 1 cup Cherries- Frozen
- 1 cup plain Greek yogurt

Directions:

1. Prepare a smooth blend of soaked oats, frozen cherries, yogurt, chia seeds, almond butter, and vanilla extract. Pour the mixture into two bowls.
2. In each bowl, add equal parts of hemp seeds, sliced almonds, and fresh berries.

BROCCOLI & SAUSAGE OMELET

Preparation Time: 10 minutes

Cooking Time: 10 minutes

Servings: 2

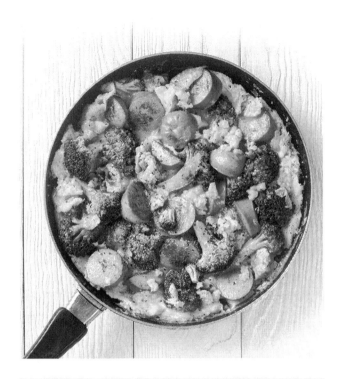

3. Pour the egg mixture over—Cook for 2 minutes per side. Run a spatula around the edges of the omelet, slide it onto a platter. Serve topped with parsley.

Sausage Quiche with Tomatoes

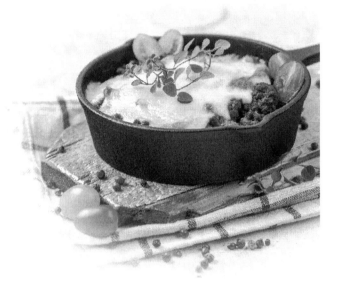

Nutrition:

- Cal 258;
- Net Carbs 3.5g;
- Fat 22g;
- Protein 12g

Ingredients:

4 eggs

2 cups pre-cooked broccoli, chopped

4 oz. sausages, sliced

4 tbsp. ricotta cheese

6 oz. roasted squash

2 tbsp. olive oil

Salt and black pepper to taste

Fresh parsley to garnish

Directions:

1. Beat eggs in a bowl, season with salt and pepper, and stir in broccoli and ricotta. In another bowl, mash the squash.

2. Add the squash to the egg mixture. Heat 1 tbsp. Of olive oil in a pan and cook sausages for 5 minutes. Drizzle the remaining olive oil.

Preparation Time: 15 minutes
Cooking Time: 10 minutes
Servings: 6

Nutrition:

- Cal 340;
- Net Carbs 3g;
- Fat 28g;
- Protein 1.7g

Ingredients:

6 eggs

12 oz. raw sausage rolls

10 cherry tomatoes, halved

2 tbsp. heavy cream

2 tbsp. Parmesan, grated

Salt and black pepper to taste

2 tbsp. parsley, chopped

5 eggplant slices

Directions:

1. Preheat the oven to 370 F. Chop the sausage rolls into the bottom of a greased pan and the eggplant slices on top of the sausage.
2. Bake for 10 minutes, then leave to rest for a few minutes.
3. Complete with the cherry tomatoes. Beat the eggs together with the cream, Parmesan, salt, and pepper.
4. Pour the egg mixture over the sausage. Bake for about 20 minutes. Serve sprinkled with parsley.

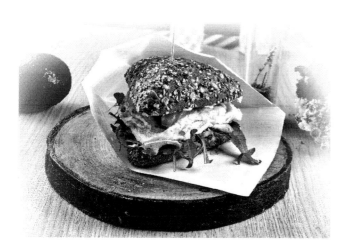

FITNESS BURGER WITH OMELET AND SALMON

Preparation Time: 10 minutes
Cooking Time: 6 minutes
Servings: 2

Nutrition:
- Cal 514;
- Net Carbs 5.8g;
- Fat 47g;
- Protein 37g

Ingredients:
1 cup rocket

2 loaves of wholemeal flour
2 tbsp. chopped chives
2 oz. smoked salmon, sliced
1 spring onion, sliced
4 eggs, beaten
3 tbsp. cream cheese
1 teaspoon linseed oil
Salt and black pepper to taste

Directions:

1. In a small bowl, combine the chives and cream cheese; set aside. Season the eggs with salt and pepper. Melt butter in a pan and add the eggs; cook for 3 minutes.
2. Flip the omelet over and cook for another 2 minutes until golden.
3. Place them on the bread and spread the chive mixture. Complete with salmon and onion slices. Cover with another slice of bread and serve.

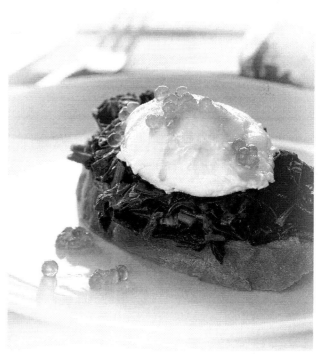

POACHED EGG WITH SPINACH

Preparation time: 5 minutes
Cooking time: 5 minutes
Servings: 1

Nutrition:
- calories 200,
- fat 8g,
- fiber 2g,
- carbs 8g,
- protein 6g

Ingredients:

1 tablespoon. rice vinegar

2 egg

2 slices of soy bread

2 tbsp lumpfish roe

2 cups of spinach

1 tbsp extra virgin olive oil

Salt

Black pepper.

Directions:

1. Put some water in a saucepan and heat.
2. Simmer, add vinegar, and mix.
3. Break the egg into boiling water and cook for 4 minutes, making sure it stays in a compact form.
4. Heat the oil in a saucepan and cook the spinach with the lid on 5 min.
5. Toast the bread.
6. Put the slices of bread on the plate and place the well-squeezed spinach on top.
4. Transfer the egg to the slices of bread and sprinkle with the lumpfish eggs. Serve for breakfast.

Eggs and Salsa

Preparation time: 5 minutes

Cooking time: 5 minutes

Servings: 4

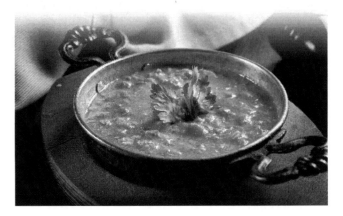

Nutrition:
- calories 340,
- fat 14g,
- fiber 4g,
- carbs 3g,
- protein 5g,

Ingredients:

- 1 red pepper, chopped
- 1 cups tomatoes sauce
- 1 green onion (bunch)
- 1 bunch cilantro, chopped
- 1 cup red onion, chopped
- Juice from 1 lime
- 2 small habanero chilies, chopped
- 2 garlic cloves, minced
- 4 eggs, whisked
- A drizzle of olive oil
- Sea salt

Directions:

1. Mix the tomatoes, green onions, red onion, habanero, garlic, cilantro, lime juice, and mix well.
2. Heat a pan with a drizzle of oil, add the eggs and mix for 2 minutes

3. Add a pinch of salt and pour the mixture of tomato and vegetables.
4. Cook for another 5min.
5. Divide and serve on plates, add fresh cilantro and serve.

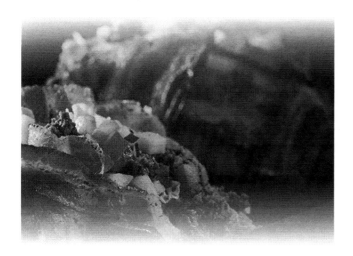

Bacon tacos

Preparation time: 10 minutes
Cooking time: 20 minutes
Servings: 4

Nutrition:
- calories 260,
- fat 8g,
- fiber 2g,
- carbs 8g,

Ingredients
Fourteen pieces halved bacon
An avocado seeded, peeled and sliced
Black pepper powder quarter tsp.
Monterey jack shredded in half a cup
Five eggs
Fresh chives chopped two tbsp.
Almond milk one tbsp.
A pinch of salt
Unsweetened butter one tbsp.
A little hot sauce

Directions
1. Begin by preparing the taco shells first.
2. Heat the oven in advance at 400c.
3. Get a baking sheet and line the inside with foil. Place the bacon strips in it, crisscrossing each other to form a square at the end. Do this again to form three consecutive weaves.
4. Take the black pepper powder and season the arranged bacon pieces and press flat the bacon using a baking rack that is inverted.
5. Place the sheet for baking in the oven that you heated in advance and let the bacon bake until it is crispy, which will take half an hour.
6. When the bacon is ready, using a knife for paring, cut up the crispy bacon squares to form small circles, which will be the taco shells. This should be done very fast.
7. Get the eggs and crack them in a mixing container. Add the almond milk and whisk both until they are well mixed.
8. Take a frying pan and over medium heat melt the unsweetened butter.
9. Follow this by pouring the whisked egg mixture and slowly move the eggs around to turn them into scrambled eggs. Add salt and black pepper powder for seasoning followed by chives then remove the frying pan from the heat.
10. Get a plate that you will use to serve and arrange the bacon taco shells on top of it.
11. Add the scrambled eggs on top of the bacon taco shells, then add a little cheese, avocado slices, and a little hot sauce as well.

Delicious Shakshuka

Preparation time: 10 minutes
Cooking time: 30 minutes
Servings: 4

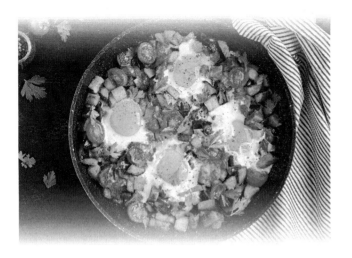

Nutrition:
- calories 40,
- fat 1g,
- fiber 2g,
- carbs 8g,
- protein 2g

Ingredients

Feta cheese crumbled half a cup

Eggplant cut into cubes, half a cup

Sliced courgette, half a cup

Two tablespoons extra virgin olive oil.

Four eggs

One sliced onion

Black pepper powder one teaspoon.

Sliced red sweet peppers

A quarter of a teaspoon of salt.

Three minced garlic cloves

Red pepper flakes half a teaspoon.

Three pureed tomatoes

Coriander half a teaspoon.

Ground cumin two tsp.

Paprika a teaspoon.

Fresh chopped parsley a teaspoon.

Pieces of almond bread

Directions

1. Preheat the oven to 375 ° C.
2. Heat the olive oil in a large skillet over medium heat.
3. Add the sliced onion and let it fry until it has a nice golden color. Complete with the pieces of red pepper, aubergine, zucchini, and cook until the peppers are soft.
4. Also, add the minced garlic cloves to this mixture and cook until the garlic is nice and fragrant.
5. Add the sliced tomato, cumin powder, coriander, paprika, and red pepper flakes. Also, add the salt and black pepper powder. Let this mixture cook for ten minutes until it thickens.
6. Take a large pan and pour in the cooked sauce. With a spoon, make eight holes in the sauce and each slot an egg and pour it.
7. Sprinkle some salt and pepper on the eggs for seasoning. Using aluminum foil, cover the pan and transfer it to the oven that you previously heated for a quarter of an hour until the eggs are well cooked.
8. When they are ready, sprinkle the crumbled feta with fresh parsley.
9. Cut into slices and serve with the almond bread.

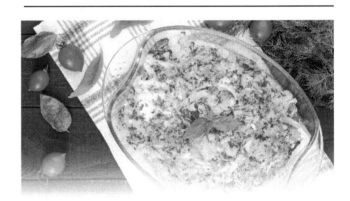

EGGS WITH CAULIFLOWER

Preparation time: 10 min
Cooking time: 20 min
Servings: 4

Nutrition:
- calories 40,
- fat 1g,
- fiber 2g,
- carbs 8g,
- protein 2g

Ingredients

A medium head of pre-cooked cauliflower (Boil for 20 min)

One tablespoon extra virgin olive oil.

Three eggs

A quarter of a teaspoon of freshly ground black pepper.

A quarter of a teaspoon of salt.

Cheddar cheese shredded a cup.

Four slices of sliced bacon

Paprika two tsp.

Fresh chives a teaspoon.

Directions

1. Place the shredded cauliflower in a container, add the eggs and shredded cheddar cheese, and salt. Mix them well.
2. Take a large skillet and heat the olive oil over medium heat. Fry the bacon until it becomes crisp.
3. Mix with the mixture.
4. Preheat the oven to 400 F.
5. Take a baking sheet, pour the contents, and let it cook for 20 min.
6. Sprinkle the paprika and chives and serve.

BACON WITH BRUSSELS SPROUTS AND EGGS

Preparation time: 20 min

Cooking time: 10 min

Servings: 4

Nutrition:
- calories 100,
- fat 7g,
- fiber 2g,
- carbs 8g,
- protein 6g

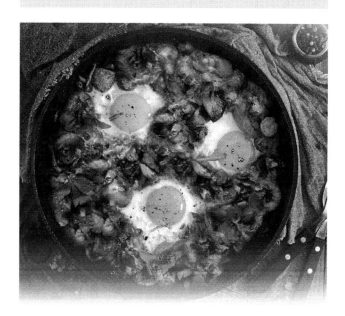

Ingredients

- 4 eggs large
- Trimmed and halved Brussels sprouts one cup
- Quarter tsp. black pepper freshly ground
- Bacon six slices
- Salt quarter tsp.
- Olive oil extra virgin two tbsp.
- Buffalo sauce three tbsp.
- Flakes of red pepper quarter tsp.
- Powder of garlic half tsp.
- Fresh chives chopped one tsp.

Directions

1. Heat your oven in advance at 425c.
2. Get a mixing container and in it mix the halved Brussels sprouts, powder of garlic, flakes of red pepper, bacon, buffalo sauce, and olive oil.
3. Add the black pepper that has been freshly ground and the salt to season the mix.
4. Get a large baking sheet and cover it with the mixture evenly.

5. Place the large baking sheet into the oven you heated in advance and let it bake for fifteen minutes when the bacon will be crispy and the Brussels sprouts tender.

6. Take the sheet out and use a wooden spoon to make six holes in the baked mixture.

7. Crack the eggs and pour in the holes you made using the wooden spoon and sprinkle a little black pepper that has been freshly ground and salt to season the eggs.

8. Return the baking sheet into the oven and bake for ten minutes until the eggs are done. Take the baking sheet out of the oven and sprinkle the fresh chives and buffalo sauce on top before serving.

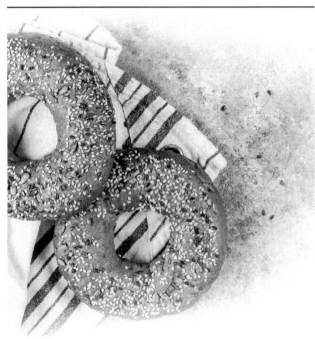

LOW CARB BAGELS

Preparation time: 10 minutes
Cooking time: 20 minutes
Servings: 4
Nutrition:
- calories 270,
- fat 18g,
- fiber 1g,
- carbs 3g,
- protein 22g

Ingredients
- Almond flour two cups
- Bagel seasoning three tbsp.
- Powder for baking one tbsp.
- Three eggs
- Mozzarella cheese shredded three cups
- Cream cheese quarter a cup

Directions
1. Heat your oven in advance at 400c.
2. Get two baking sheets and line them well with paper made from parchment.
3. Get a large mixing container and in it, mix the almond flour with the powder for baking.
4. Mix the mozzarella cheese and the cream cheese in a bowl that can be used in a microwave. Place the bowl in a microwave for two minutes when the cheese melts and combines.
5. Get the mixture of cheese from the bowl once out of the microwave and pour it into the mixing container with the flour from almonds and the powder for baking. Mix all the ingredients until well mixed.
6. Take the dough when done and divide it into eight parts that are equal in measure. Using your palms, take each of the eight dough parts and roll them into balls.
7. Using your fingers, create a hole in each of the balls, and gently stretch the dough to form the shape of a bagel.
8. Take one egg and beat it in a bowl. Brush the eggs on top of each made bagel following this by sprinkling the bagel seasoning at the top as well.
9. Place the bagel dough in the oven on its rack, which is in the middle for twenty-five minutes when they are nice and golden in color.

10. Remove the bagels from the oven and let them get cold for about ten minutes before serving them.

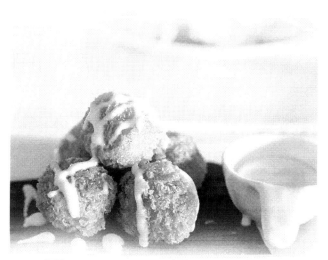

Homemade Tuna Fish Cakes with Lemon Sauce

Preparation time: 10 minutes
Cooking time: 20 minutes
Servings: 1

Nutrition:
- calories 350,
- fat 8g,
- fiber 2g,
- carbs 8g,
- protein 26g

Ingredients

For the tuna cakes:
- Half a zucchini, grated
- 1 can of drained tuna
- 2 tbsp oats
- 2 tbsp cheese, shredded
- 1 egg
- 0.24 tsp garlic salt
- 0.25 tsp dill
- 0.25 tsp onion powder

For the sauce:
- 2 tbsp yogurt, Greek-style is best
- 1 tsp juice of a lemon
- 0.25 tsp dill
- 0.25 tsp garlic salt

Direction

1. Take a piece of cheesecloth, or similar and place the grated zucchini inside, twisting so that all the liquid comes out
2. In a medium bowl, place the drained zucchini inside and add the tuna, oats, shredded cheese, the garlic salt, dill, onion powder, pepper, and the egg, combining everything together well
3. Take a large frying pan and add a little olive oil, or cooking spray if you prefer
4. Take half of the mixture and form a ball, before flattening it into a fish cake style, repeating with the other half
5. Place the cakes into the frying pan, cooking over medium heat for around 6 minutes on each side
6. Meanwhile, combine the sauce ingredients into a small mixing bowl and ensure they are mixed together well
7. Once the fish cakes are cooked place them on a serving plate and allow to cool just slightly
8. Add a spoonful of the sauce on top and enjoy!

Healthy Breakfast Burritos

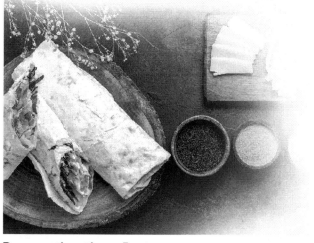

Preparation time: 5 minutes
Cooking time: 10 minutes
Servings: 5

Nutrition:
- calories 350,
- fat 8g,
- fiber 2g,
- carbs 8g,
- protein 26g

Ingredients

8 eggs

1 tbsp milk

1 tbsp garlic, minced

1 red pepper, minced

Half an onion,
   (red if possible, minced)

4 slices of bacon, cooked

Salt

Pepper

4 tortilla wraps
   (multi-grain or wholegrain)

A little cheese (optional)

Direction

1. Take a medium-sized saucepan and heat over a medium heat
2. Add the garlic and cook for a couple of minutes, until fragrant
3. Whisk the eggs with the milk and place to one side
4. Add the pepper and onion to the pan and allow to cook for a couple more minutes,
5. Add the eggs to the pan and cook for 4 minutes
6. Once cooked, add a quarter of the egg mixture onto each tortilla wrap and add one piece of the bacon on top
7. You can add cheese if you want, although it isn't necessary
8. Wrap up and enjoy!

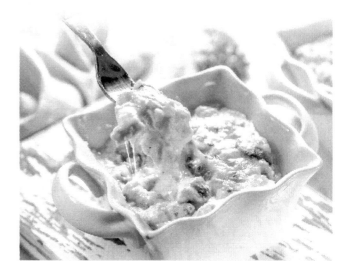

DELICIOUS EGG CASSEROLE

Preparation time: 10 minutes

Cooking time: 30 minutes

Servings: 6

Nutrition:
- calories 200,
- fat 8g,
- fiber 2g,
- carbs 8g,
- protein 6g

Ingredients

4.5 cups brown bread, cut into cubes

2 cups cheese, shredded

10 eggs, beaten

0.25-pint milk

1 tsp dry mustard

1 tsp salt

0/25 tsp onion powder

8 slices bacon, cooked and crumbled up

0.5 cup mushrooms, chopped

Direction

1. Preheat your oven to 325C

2. Take a baking dish, around 13 inches in size and spray it with some cooking spray, to avoid sticking
3. Take the cubed pieces of bread and lay them in the bottom of the baking dish, evenly, so that the bottom is totally covered over
4. Add the cheese on the top, in one even layer
5. Take a separate mixing bowl and combine the milk, mustard, eggs, pepper, onion powder and the salt until completely mixed together
6. Add the mixture over the top of the bread and the cheese evenly
7. Now add the bacon and mushrooms on top, again making sure to stick to an even layer
8. Place the baking dish in the oven for half an hour. You will know when it is finished because it will have turned a wonderful golden brown
9. Remove from the oven and place to one side

- calories 275,
- fat 20g,
- fiber 2g,
- carbs 8g,
- protein 20g

Ingredients:

- 2 cups short grain brown rice, rinsed
- 6 green tea bags
- ½ cup brown lentils, rinsed
- 12 cups water
- Salt to taste

Direction:

1. Add all the ingredients into a Dutch oven. Cover with the lid.
2. Discard tea bags.
3. Ladle into bowls. Serve with any of the optional toppings.

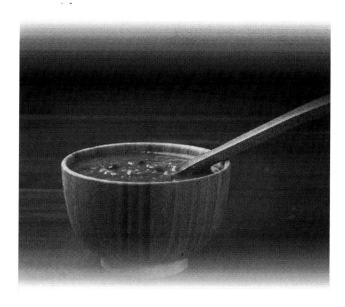

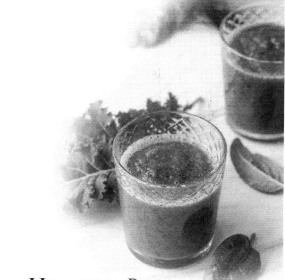

HEALTHY BREAKFAST SMOOTHIE

Preparation Time: 5 Minutes
Cooking Time: 1 Minute
Servings: 1

Nutrition:

- Calories: 117,
- Fat: 15 g

BROWN RICE, LENTILS AND GREEN TEA PORRIDGE

Preparation time: 10 minutes
Cooking time: 20 minutes
Servings: 8
Nutrition:

- Protein: 20 g
- Carbs: 5 g

Ingredients:

1 ¼ cups coconut milk, or almond or regular dairy milk

½ cup kale or spinach, or both (¼ Cup each) if you prefer

½ avocado, sliced into smaller pieces

¾ cup cucumber, sliced into smaller pieces

1 cup of green grapes

¼ teaspoon ginger, peeled and grated

1 scoop Plant-based protein powder

Honey to taste

Directions:

1. Add all of these ingredients into your blender in the order they appear above.
2. Blend them until the mixture is smooth
3. Taste it and add as much honey as you desire
4. Pour into a glass and serve.

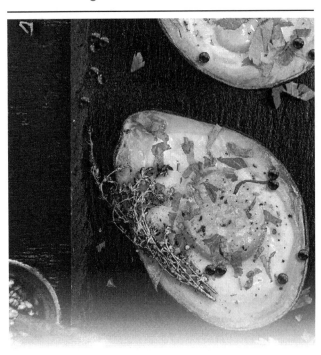

AVOCADO EGG BOWLS

Preparation Time: 10 minutes

Cooking Time: 40 minutes

Servings: 3

Nutrition:
- Calories 215,
- Fat 18 g
- Carbs 8 g
- Fiber 2.6 g
- Protein 9 g

Ingredients:
- Coconut oil- 1 Teaspoon
- Organic, free-range eggs-2
- Salt and pepper- to sprinkle
- Large & ripe avocado- 1

For Garnishing:
- Chopped walnuts, as many as you like
- Balsamic Pearls
- Fresh thyme

Directions:

1. Slice your avocado in two, then take out the pit and remove enough of the inside so that there is enough space inside to accommodate an entire egg.
2. Cut off a little bit of the bottom of the avocado so that the avocado will sit upright as you place it on a stable surface.
3. Open your eggs and put each of the yolks in a separate bowl or container. Place the egg whites in the same small bowl. Sprinkle some pepper and salt to the whites, according to your personal taste, then mix them well.
4. Melt the coconut oil in a pan that has a lid that fits and put it on med-high.
5. Put in the avocado boats, with the meaty side down on the pan, the skin side up and sauté them for approx. 35 seconds, or when they become darker in color.
6. Turn them over, then add to the spaces inside, almost filling the inside with the whites of the eggs.

7. Then, reduce the temperature and place the lid. Let them sit covered it for approx. 16 to 20 minutes until the whites are just about fully cooked.

8. Gently add one yolk onto each of the avocados and keep cooking them for 4 to 5 minutes, just until they get to the point of cook you want them at.

9. Move the avocados to a dish and add toppings to each of them using the walnuts, the balsamic pearls, or/and thyme.

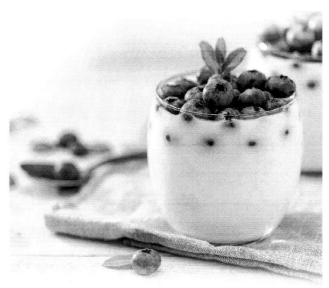

BLUEBERRIES BREAKFAST BOWL

Preparation Time: 35 minutes

Cooking Time: 0 minutes

Servings: 1

Nutrition:
- Calories: 202,
- Fat: 16.8 g
- Protein: 10.2 g
- Carbs: 9.8 g
- Fiber: 5.8 g

- **Ingredients:**
- 1 teaspoon chia seeds
- 1 cup almond milk
- ¼ cup of fresh blueberries or fresh fruits
- 1 pack sweetener for taste

Directions:

1. Mix the chia seeds with almond milk. Stir periodically.

2. Place in the fridge to cool for 30 minutes, and then serve with fresh fruit. Enjoy!

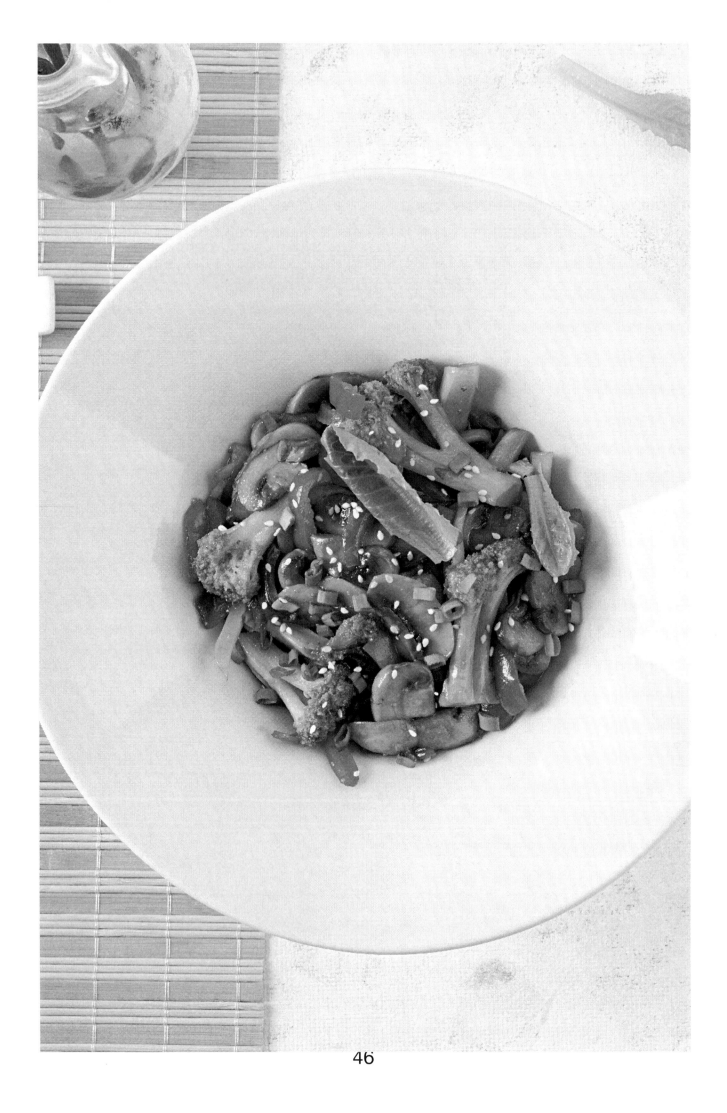

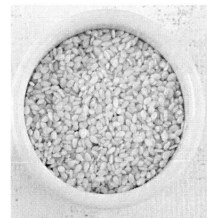
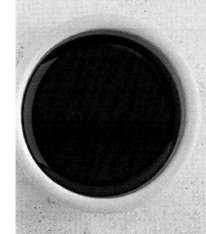

A Bit of Lunch Cuisine in Between

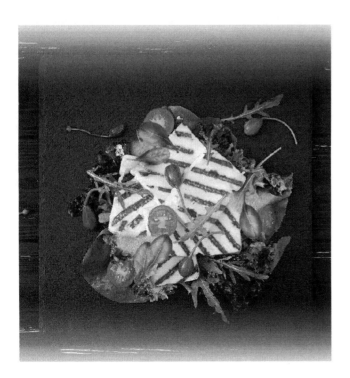

CITRUS AND HALLOUMI SALAD

Preparation time: 10 minutes

Cooking time: 15 minutes

Servings: 4

Nutrition:

- calories 282,
- fat 4g,
- fiber 2g,
- carbs 14g,
- protein 3g

Ingredients

- 2 oranges
- 1.5 tbsp mustard, wholegrain works best
- 1.5 tsp honey
- 3 tbsp olive oil plus and an extra tbsp for cooking
- 1 tbsp white wine vinegar
- 2 carrots, peeled and cut into thin slices using a grater
- 1 x 225g of halloumi, cut into slices
- A handful of baby spinach or watercress

Direction

1. Take the oranges and cut away the peel and the pith, cutting into segments, maintaining the juice in the bowl, and placing the segments to one side
2. Add the mustard, oil, vinegar and the honey and combine, seasoning a little if need be
3. Toss the carrots in the mixture
4. Take a medium-sized frying pan and add a little oil, over a medium heat
5. Cook the halloumi on both sides until golden, for a few minutes
6. Meanwhile, toss the baby spinach or the watercress in the mixture and arrange on a plate
7. Add the halloumi on top and pour the mixture over the cheese, adding the oranges on the side

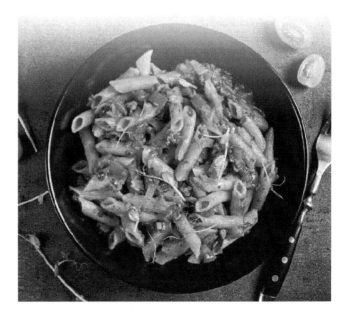

PASTA BOLOGNESE

Preparation time: 10 minutes

Cooking time: 35 minutes

Servings: 5

Nutrition:

- calories 182,

- fat 4g,
- fiber 2g,
- carbs 14g,
- protein 3g

Ingredients

2 tsp olive oil

3 onions, chopped finely

2 carrots, peeled and chopped finely

2 celery stick, chopped finely

3 cloves of garlic, chopped finely

250g of lean steak/beef mince

500g tomatoes pasta

1 tbsp vegetable stock

1 tsp paprika, smoked works well

4 pieces of thyme, fresh

100mg penne, wholemeal

45g parmesan cheese, grated finely

Direction

1. Take a large pan and add the oil, heat over a medium heat
2. Add the onions and cook until translucent
3. Add the carrots, garlic, and celery, cooking for 5 minutes
4. Add the mince to the pan and break it up well
5. Once the mince has browned, add the stock and the passata, adding 1 liter of hot water
6. Stir well and then add the thyme and paprika, combining once more
7. Add the lid to the pan and allow to simmer for 15 minutes
8. Add the penne and stir through, cooking for another 165 minutes
9. Add the cheese and stir
10. Serve in bowls whilst still warm.

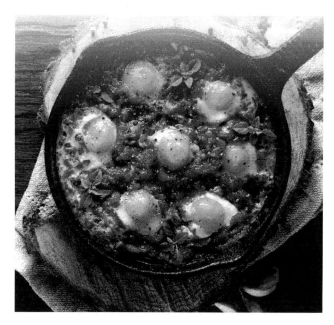

Eggs with Chilli and Red Beans

Preparation time: 5 minutes

Cooking time: 5 minutes

Servings: 3

Nutrition:

- calories 550,
- fat 16g,
- fiber 32g,
- carbs 18g,
- protein 43g

Ingredients

- 2 teaspoons of olive oil
- 1 red chilli, thinly sliced
- 1 clove of garlic, sliced
- 6 eggs
- 1 x 500g can of red beans, not drained
- 1 x 400 g can of tomatoes, possibly cherry tomatoes
- 0.25 teaspoons of cumin seeds
- A little coriander, chopped

Direction

1. Take a large skillet and add the oil, letting it warm over medium-high heat

2. Add the garlic and chilli and cook until soft

3. Add the entire contents of the can of beans to the pan, along with the tomatoes, mixing thoroughly

4. Add the cumin seeds

5. Cook everything for 15 min

6. Carefully break the eggs into the pan, cook covered for 2 min

7. After a few minutes, remove the pan and add some cilantro

8. Serve still hot!

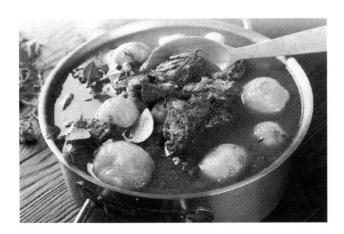

Potato and Beef Soup

Preparation time: 10 minutes
Cooking time: 60 minutes
Servings: 6
Nutrition:
- calories 555,
- fat 28g,
- fiber 2g,
- carbs 6g,
- protein 67g

Ingredients:
Cooking spray
Cumin (0.5 tsp.)
Chopped cilantro (2 tbsps.)
Red or Yukon Gold potatoes (1.5 cup)
Water (1.5 cup)
Diced tomatoes (2 cup)
Diced onion (1 pc.)
Beef sirloin steak (0.5 lb.)

Directions

1. Rinse off the beef steak and blot it dry. Slice into smaller cubes and set aside.

2. Coat the inside of a heavy stew pot with some cooking spray and place on the hot stove for about a minute to heat-up the pot.

3. Add in the prepared beef to the stew pot and cook until the pieces are browned all over. This will take about five minutes. Stir in the onion and let it cook until tender.

4. Stir in the water, cumin, and tomatoes. Mix this well and bring it to a boil. Once at a boil, reduce the heat to medium, and cover and let simmer for about 20 minutes.

5. Uncover the pot and then stir in the cubed potatoes. Cover this and let it simmer for a bit longer until both the beef and the potatoes are tender, which will take another 10 minutes.

6. At this time, turn the heat off and let it stand, with the cover on, for about 5 minutes.

7. Ladle this into some soup bowls and then serve.

Lemon Pangasius

Preparation time: 10 minutes
Cooking time: 10 minutes
Servings: 6

Nutrition:
- calories 300,
- fat 8g,
- fiber 2g,
- carbs 8g,
- protein 23g

Ingredients:

Boiled asparagus (0.25 cup)

Diced carrots (0.25 cup)

Chicken broth (0.75 cup)

Red onion, sliced (0.5)

Pangasius fillet cut in half (0.5 lbs)

Dill, dried (0.25 tsp)

Lemon dressing (1 tsp)

Cornstarch (1 tablespoon)

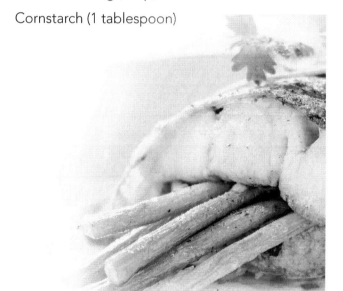

Directions

1. To get started with this recipe, take a pan and place it on the stovetop. Pour in the chicken stock before adding the lemon dressing, dill, and sliced onion.

2. Cover and simmer for another 3 minutes until the onion is tender.

3. Uncover the pan and add the asparagus, corn and diced carrots. Place the flounder on top of the other ingredients and simmer for another 5 minutes so that the fish can cook completely.

4. Move the fish to a bowl using a slotted spoon and then cover to keep warm.

5. Remove some broth from the soup and add it to the bowl. Stir in the cornstarch before returning it to the pan. Stir well and bring to a boil.

6. Pour the broth and vegetables on the plate, place the fish on top and then serve.

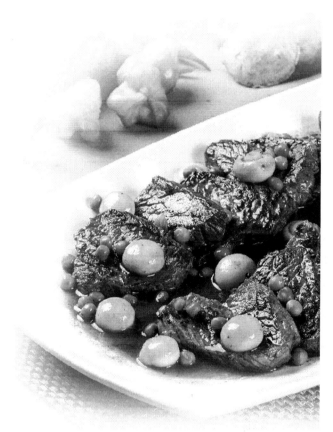

Pork Carnitas

Preparation time: 10 minutes

Cooking time: 50 minutes

Servings: 2

Nutrition:
- calories 294,
- fat 12g,
- fiber 2g,
- carbs 8g,
- protein 45g

Ingredients:
- Pepper
- Salt (0.25 tsp.)

- Sweet and sour mushrooms (1 cup)
- Dark molasses (0.5 tbsp.)
- Orange juice (0.5 tbsp.)
- Brown sugar (1 tbsp.)
- Minced garlic clove (1 pc.)
- Pork tenderloin (0.5 lb.)

Directions

1. Rinse off the pork tenderloin and blot it down with some paper towels. Slice thinly and then set it aside.

2. Place a skillet on a flame or burner set to high, and then heat it up for about a minute. Once the skillet is hot, add the pork tenderloin. Cook these for about 4 minutes until the pork is tender and cooked throughout.

3. Drain out the oil before stirring in the pepper, salt, molasses, orange juice, mushrooms and brown sugar.

4. Stir this around and simmer until your sauce is thick. Turn off the heat and let it stand for a few minutes to thicken before serving.

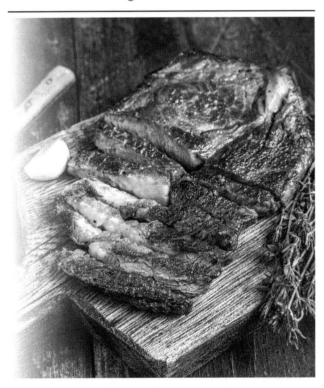

GRILLED STEAK SALAD

Preparation time: 10 minutes
Cooking time: 60 minutes

Nutrition:
- calories 540,
- fat 8g,
- fiber 2g,
- carbs 8g,
- protein 67g

Ingredients:

Cucumber, sliced (1 pc.)

Halved cherry tomatoes (1 cup)

Mixed greens (1 package)

Flank steak (1 lb.)

Soy sesame dressing

Grated carrot (1 pc.)

Directions

1. Take out a bowl and add in the steak with a drizzle of the dressing. Make sure that all your steak is well coated with the dressing and then set aside for a minimum of 30 minutes to marinate.

2. After the steak has had some time to marinate, turn on the grill, and get it preheated to medium-high. Remove the excess dressing and place the steak on the grill.

3. Let the steak grill until it reaches 145 degrees, which will take about 5 minutes on each side. Move the steak to a plate and allow the steak to rest for at least 5 minutes before slicing. Cutting the stake too soon will ruin the steak! Letting it rest is important to a juicy steak.

4. Plate your veggies first as the base of the bowl, then layer the steak over-top. Drizzle with some of the dressing and then serve.

TURKEY WALNUT SALAD

Preparation time: 10 min
Cooking time: 20 min

Nutrition:
- calories 390,
- fat 4g,
- fiber 2g,
- carbs 8g,
- protein 56g

Ingredients:

Chopped walnuts (0.25 cup)

Chopped celery (1 pc.)

Chopped yellow onion (0.5 pc.)

Minced turkey (8 oz.)

Pepper

Salt

Parsley (2 tsp.)

Lemon juice (1 tsp.)

Dijon mustard (1 tbsp.)

Greek yogurt (2 tbsps.)

Mayo (2 tbsps.)

Dried cranberries (3 tbsps.)

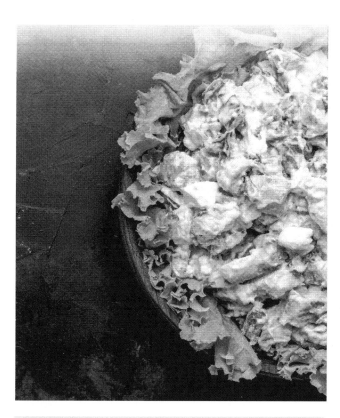

Directions

1. Take out a bowl and combine the cranberries, walnuts, celery, onion, and turkey.

2. In another bowl, combine the pepper, salt, parsley, lemon juice, mustard, Greek yogurt, and mayo.

3. Combine both bowls together and toss well to mix evenly before serving.

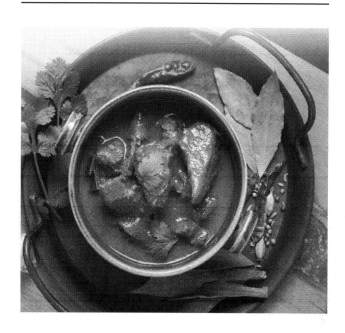

LAMB CURRY

Preparation time: 10 minutes

Cooking time: 4 hours

Servings: 6

Nutrition:
- calories 181,
- fat 9g,
- fiber 5g,
- carbs 8g,
- protein 14g

Ingredients:

Fresh ginger – 2 tbsp. grated

Garlic – 2 cloves, peeled and minced

Cardamom – 2 tsp

Onion – 1 peeled and hopped

Cloves – 6

Lamb meat – 1 pound, cubed

Cumin powder – 2 tsp

Garam masala – 1 tsp

Chilli powder – ½ tsp

Turmeric – 1 tsp

Coriander – 2 tsp

Spinach – 1 pound

Canned – 14 ounces

Directions:

1. In a slow cooker, mix lamb with tomatoes, spinach, ginger, garlic, onion, cardamom, cloves, cumin, garam masala, chilli, turmeric, and coriander.

2. Stir well. Cover and cook on high for 4 hours.

3. Uncover slow cooker, stir the chilli, divide into bowls, and serve.

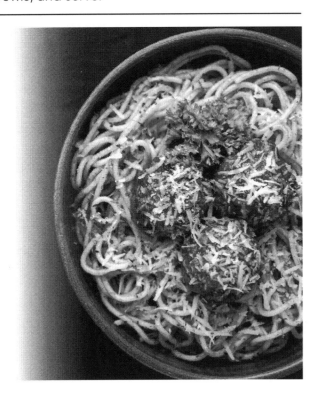

Meaty Spaghetti Squash

Preparation time: 10 minutes

Cooking time: 50 minutes

Servings: 6

Nutrition:
- calories 210g,
- fat 12g,
- fiber 2g,
- carbs 8g,
- protein 6g

Ingredients

An egg

Oregano dried one tsp.

Basil dried one tsp.

Parmesan cheese quarter cup grated

Salt half a tsp.

Minced beef four cups

Worcestershire sauce one tsp.

Marinara sauce low carb three cups

Mozzarella cheese two cups shredded

Low carb cooked spaghetti squash four cups

Directions

1. Heat your oven in advance at 250c.

2. Take a mixing container and in it mix the minced beef, Worcestershire sauce, basil dried, oregano dried, egg, salt, and parmesan cheese grated.

3. Take small scoops of the mix and make balls of meat taking care because they will be very soft.

4. Take a sheet used for baking and coat its bottom with a quarter cup of the marinara sauce. Arrange the balls of meat you have prepared at the top then pour the remaining marinara sauce at the top coating all of them.

5. Place the sheet for baking in the oven you had heated in advance and let the balls of meat bake for half an hour until well cooked.

6. After half an hour, sprinkle the shredded mozzarella cheese on top of the baked balls of meat then replace it in the oven for the cheese to melt for about three minutes.

7. When all the cheese has melted, take them out of the oven and allow them to get cold completely before serving.

8. Take a plate and in it, place the spaghetti squash and scoops of the baked balls of meat and enjoy.

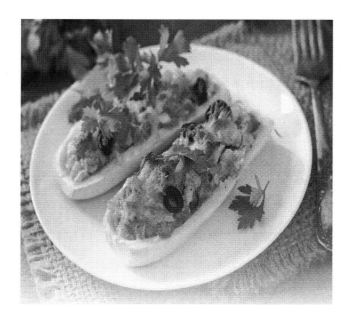

Parmesan Chicken with Zucchini

Preparation time: 10 min
Cooking time: 20 min
Servings: 6

Nutrition:
calories 267,
fat 34g,
fiber 2g,
carbs 8g,

Ingredients
Minced chicken two cups
Big zucchinis four halved along their length
Low carb tomato basil sauce
Olive oil extra virgin three tbsp.
Black olives quarter cup
Parmesan cheese quarter cup grated
Small Yellow onion diced
Mozzarella cheese quarter cup grated
Two garlic cloves minced
Basil dried one tsp.
Quarter tsp. salt
Quarter tsp. black pepper powder freshly ground

Directions
1. Heat your oven in advance at 400c.
2. Get a large pan used for baking and coat its bottom with the low carb tomato basil sauce.
3. Get a melon scooper and with care, scoop out the flesh of the zucchini. Take this flesh and blend it gently in a blender.
4. Take a large pan used for frying and add olive oil extra virgin in it. Heat the oil over medium heat and when it is hot, add in the diced yellow onion. Let the onion fry for three minutes, then add in the minced garlic and cook this for one minute until the garlic is fragrant.
5. Pour in the minced chicken and the blended flesh of zucchini. Season this with the black pepper powder freshly ground and salt. Cover and let this cook for five minutes until the chicken is well cooked. Pour out the excess fluid that may remain after the chicken is cooked.
6. Take a little of the sauce and pour it into the cooked chicken stirring so that it covers all the chicken. Let this mixture simmer over medium heat for around eight minutes.
7. Take the zucchini that has been halved and scooped and place them on a plate. Scoop the minced chicken mixture and place it in the middle of the halved zucchini. Take the stuffed zucchini pieces and place them on the dish for baking you prepared earlier.
8. Cover the dish with foil and place it in the oven you had heated in advance. Let them bake in the oven for twenty-five minutes when the zucchini softens.
9. When the zucchini is soft, take the dish for baking from the oven and unwrap the foil. Sprinkle the grated parmesan, olives, and mozzarella cheese at the top. Put back the dish for baking in the oven and let it bake until all the cheese melts well.
10. Take it from the oven and serve.

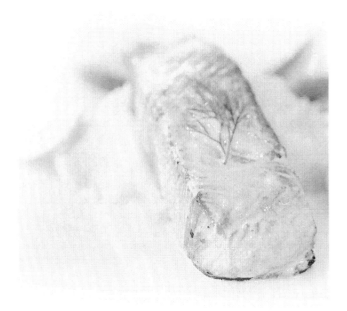

Lemon Baked Salmon

Preparation Time: 5 minutes

Cooking Time: 20 minutes

Servings: 2

Nutrition:
- calories 571,
- fat 44g,
- fiber 2g,
- carbs 2g,
- protein 42g

Ingredients:

12 oz. filets of salmon

2 lemons, sliced thinly

2 tbsps. Olive oil

Salt and black pepper, to taste

3 sprigs thyme

1/2 cup of milk cream

Directions:

1. Preheat the oven to 350° F.
2. Place half the sliced lemons on the bottom of a baking dish.
3. Place the fillets over the lemons and cover with the remaining lemon slices and thyme.
4. Pour a drizzle of olive oil and the milk cream into the pan and cook for 20 minutes.
5. Season with salt, pepper and cooking juices.

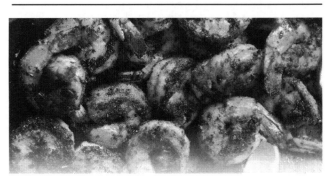

Easy Blackened Shrimp

Preparation Time: 10 min

Cooking Time: 6 min

Servings: 2

Nutrition:
- calories 152,
- fat 4g,
- fiber 1g,
- carbs 8g,
- protein 24g

Ingredients:

½ lb. shrimp, peeled and deveined

2 tbsp. blackened seasoning

1 tsp olive oil

Juice of 1 lemon

Directions:

1. Toss all ingredients (except oil) together until shrimp are well coated.
2. In a non-stick skillet, heat the oil to medium-high heat.
3. Add shrimp and cook 2-3 minutes per side.
4. Serve immediately.

Pan-Fried Cod

Preparation time: 5 minutes

Cooking time: 10 minutes

Servings: 2

Nutrition:
- calories 253,
- fat 14.3,
- fiber 0.2,
- carbs 1.2,
- protein 30.

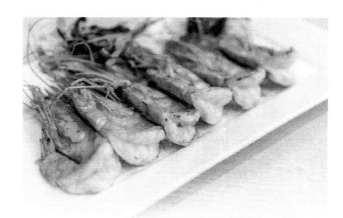

GRILLED SHRIMP EASY SEASONING

Preparation Time: 5 minutes
Cooking Time: 5 minutes
Servings: 4

Nutrition:
- calories 101,
- fat 3g,
- fiber 1g,
- carbs 1g,
- protein 28g

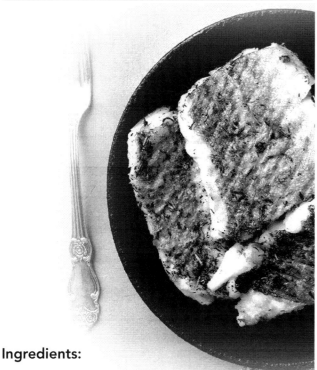

Ingredients:

Shrimp Seasoning
- 1 tsp garlic powder
- 1 tsp kosher salt
- 1 tsp Italian seasoning
- ¼ tsp cayenne pepper

Grilling
- 2 tbsps. Olive oil
- 1 tbsp. lemon juice
- 1 lb. jumbo shrimp, peeled, deveined
- Ghee for the grill

Ingredients:
- 12 oz cod fillet
- 1 tablespoon scallions, chopped
- 1 tablespoon butter
- 1 tablespoon coconut oil
- 1 teaspoon garlic, diced
- 1 teaspoon cumin seeds
- 1 teaspoon coriander seeds
- 1 teaspoon salt

Directions:

1. Place butter and coconut oil in the skillet and melt them.
2. Add garlic, cumin and coriander seeds.
3. Rub the fish fillet with salt and place it in the skillet.
4. Fry the fish for 2 minutes from each side or until it is light brown.
5. Transfer the cooked cod fillet in the plate and cut into 2 servings.

Directions:

1. Preheat the grill pan to high.
2. In a mixing bowl, stir together the seasoning ingredients.
3. Drizzle in the lemon juice and olive oil and stir.
4. Add the shrimp and toss to coat.
5. Brush the grill pan with ghee.

6. Grill the shrimp until pink, about 2-3 minutes per side.
7. Serve immediately.

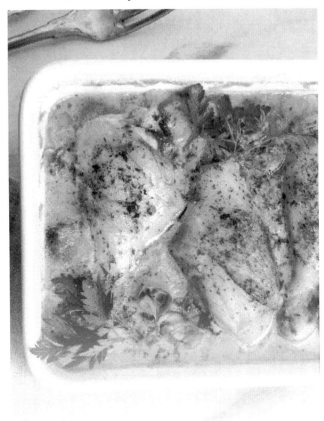

BUTTER CHICKEN

Preparation time: 5 minutes
Cooking time: 30 minutes
Servings: 4

Nutrition:
- calories 414,
- fat 9g,
- fiber 2g,
- carbs 2g,
- protein 27g

Ingredients:
- Butter – ¼ cup
- Mushrooms – 2 cups, sliced
- Chicken thighs – 4 large
- Onion powder – ½ tsp
- Garlic powder – ½ tsp
- Kosher salt – 1 tsp
- Black pepper – ¼ tsp
- Milk – ½ cup
- Dijon mustard – 1 tsp
- Fresh tarragon – 1 tbsp., chopped

Directions:
1. Season the chicken thighs with onion powder, garlic powder, salt, and pepper.
2. In a sauté pan, melt 1 tbsp. butter.
3. Sear the chicken thighs about 3 to 4 minutes per side, or until both sides are golden brown. Remove the thighs from the pan.
4. Add the remaining 3 tbsp. of butter to the pan and melt.
5. Add the mushrooms and cook for 4 to 5 minutes or until golden brown. Stirring as little as possible.
6. Add the Dijon mustard and milk to the pan. Stir to deglaze.
7. Place the chicken thighs back in the pan with the skin side up.
8. Cover and simmer for 15 minutes.
9. Stir in the fresh herbs. Let sit for 5 minutes and serve.

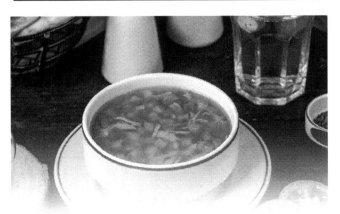

DIETER'S CHICKEN SOUP

Preparation Time: 10 min
Cooking Time: 60 min
Servings: 8

Nutrition:
- calories 200,
- fat 8g,
- fiber 2g,

- carbs 8g,
- protein 6g

Ingredients:

2 quarts sodium-free or light Chicken broth

1 pkg shredded Cabbage

2 cups Celery, diced

1 large Onion, diced

1 large Tomato, diced

2 boneless, skinless Chicken breasts, diced

1 Tablespoon ground Thyme

1 teaspoon ground sweet Basil Black pepper, to taste Mrs. Dash to taste

Direction

1. Add all ingredients to a large stock pot. Cook until tender.

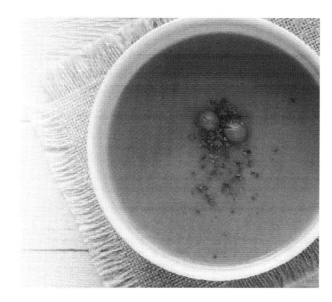

GINGERED CARROT SOUP

Preparation Time: 10 minutes
Cooking Time: 35 minutes
Servings: 5

Nutrition:
- calories 624,
- fat 8g,
- fiber 2g,
- carbs 8g,
- protein 17g

Ingredients:
- 3 Tablespoons unsalted Butter
- 1 cup Leeks, sliced (or white onion)
- 1 Tablespoon fresh Ginger, peeled and minced
- 1 ½ lbs. (~9) Carrots, peeled, cut into 1" lengths
- 2 cups Chicken stock or low-sodium Chicken broth
- 2 cups freshly squeezed Orange juice
- ¼ cup chopped fresh Mint Salt, to taste Ground white Pepper, to taste

Direction

1. In a soup pot, melt butter over medium-high heat. Add the leek and ginger, and sauté until the leek is tender but not browned (about five minutes).
2. Add the carrots, and sauté until coated with butter. Stir in the stock or broth, and bring to a boil.
3. Reduce the heat to low, cover, and simmer until the carrots are very tender (about 30 minutes).
4. Working in batches, if necessary, transfers the soup to a food processor or blender, and puree until smooth. Add the orange juice, and blend well. Stir in the chopped mint, and season to taste with salt and pepper.

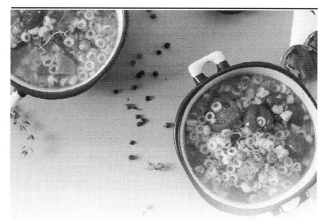

GREAT VEGETABLE SOUP

Preparation Time: 10 minutes
Cooking Time: 45 minutes
Servings: 6

Nutrition:
- calories 280,
- fat 18g,
- fiber 2g,
- carbs 18g,
- protein 10g

Ingredients:
- 1, 15-ounce can Whole Tomatoes, chopped
- 1 medium Onion, chopped
- 3 large Garlic cloves, minced
- 3-4 Celery stalks, chopped
- 1 Tablespoon dried Parsley
- 1 teaspoon dried Marjoram
- 5 cups Broccoli and other vegetables, such as: carrots, cauliflower, zucchini, peppers, leeks, potatoes, turnips, and corn.
- 6 cups Water
- 6 teaspoon low salt Bouillon or 5 Bouillon cubes, any flavor
- ½ teaspoon Black pepper
- 1 cup uncooked Macaroni or Shells Grated cheese, optional

Direction

1. In a soup pot, combine tomatoes, onion, garlic, celery, parsley and marjoram. Place over medium heat and sauté stirring frequently, until celery and onion are soft (about 20 min).
2. Watch carefully to ensure juice doesn't boil away. If it gets low, add a little water. Meanwhile, dice vegetable into half-inch cubes.
3. Add water, bouillon, vegetables, and pepper. Cover and bring to a boil. Adjust heat and simmer briskly, partially covered for 10 minutes, stirring once or twice.
4. Stir in macaroni and simmer until pasta is tender. Let rest 10 minutes, serve in soup bowls. Top with cheese

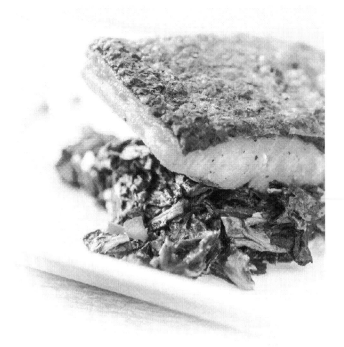

THE BEST GARLIC CILANTRO SALMON

Preparation Time: 10 min
Cooking Time: 15 min
Servings: 4

Nutrition:
- calories 140,
- fat 4g,
- fiber 2g,
- carbs 3g,
- protein 20g

Ingredients:
- 1 lb. salmon filet
- 1 tbsp. butter
- 1 lemon
- 2 cups of fresh spinach leaves
- ¼ cup fresh cilantro leaves, chopped
- 4 cloves garlic, minced
- ½ tsp kosher salt
- ½ tsp freshly cracked black pepper

Directions:

1. Preheat oven to 400° F.

2. On a foil-lined baking sheet, place salmon skin side down.
3. Squeeze lemon over the salmon.
4. Season salmon with cilantro and garlic, pepper, and salt.
5. Slice butter thinly and place pieces evenly over the salmon.
6. Bake for about 7 minutes, depending on thickness.
7. Turn the oven to broil and cook 5-7 minutes, until the top is crispy.
8. Put the spinach in a glass bowl, sprinkle with half a lemon, add 2 tbsp of water, cover with cling film, put in the microwave for 2 minutes, then lay on the plate.
9. Remove the salmon from the oven and place on the spinach, serve immediately,

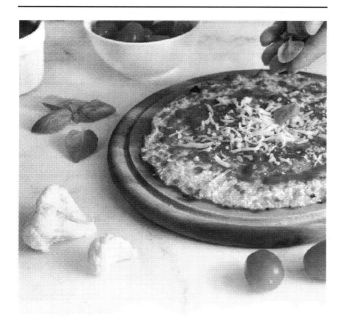

CAULIFLOWER CRUST PIZZA

Preparation Time: 20 minutes
Cooking Time: 42 minutes
Servings: 2

Nutrition:
- Calories: 119
- Fat: 6.6 g
- Carbohydrates: 8.6 g
- Fiber: 3.4 g
- Protein: 8.3 g

Ingredients:

For Crust:

1 small head cauliflower, cut into florets
2 large organic eggs, beaten lightly
½ teaspoon dried oregano
½ teaspoon garlic powder
Ground black pepper, as required

For Topping:

½ cup sugar-free pizza sauce
¾ cup mozzarella cheese, shredded
2 tablespoons Parmesan cheese, grated

Directions:

1. Preheat your oven to F 400 (200 C).
2. Line a baking sheet with a lightly greased parchment paper.
3. Add the cauliflower in a food processor and pulse until a rice-like texture is achieved.
4. In a bowl, add the cauliflower rice, eggs, oregano, garlic powder, and black pepper and mix until well combined.
5. Place the cauliflower the mixture in the center of the prepared baking sheet and with a spatula, press into a 13-inch thin circle.
6. Bake for 40 minutes or until golden brown.
7. Remove the baking sheet from the oven. Now, set the oven to broiler on high.
8. Place the tomato sauce on top of the pizza crust and with a spatula, spread evenly, and sprinkle with the cheeses.
9. Broil for about 1-2 minutes or until the cheese is bubbly and browned.
10. Remove from oven and with a pizza cutter, cut the pizza into equal-sized triangles.
11. Serve hot.

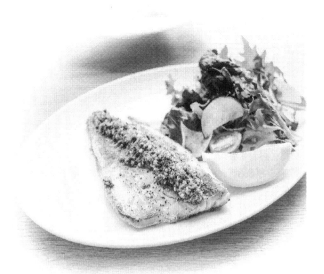

5. Lay the fillets in the mixture and top with the remaining ingredients.
6. Set under the broiler for about 7-8 minutes or until the fish breaks easily with a fork and it is not transparent.
7. Blend together the rocket, parmesan, 1 tablespoon of oil, and lemon juice. Distribute the pesto cream on fillet before serving.
8. Serve immediately.

AROMATIC DOVER SOLE FILLETS

Preparation Time: 5 minutes
Cooking Time: 20 minutes
Servings: 2

Nutrition:
- calories 244,
- fat 9g,
- fiber 2g,
- carbs 8g,
- protein 20g

Ingredients:
6 Dover Sole fillets
¼ cup virgin olive oil
The zest of 1 lemon and the juice
Dash of cardamom powder
1 cup fresh cilantro leaves
1/2 cup of Parmesan
1 cup of rocket
Pinch of sea salt

Directions:
1. Bring the fillets to room temperature.
2. Set the oven's broiler to high.
3. Pour half of the oil in an oven tray.
4. Add half of the cilantro leaves, half of the lemon zest, and the cardamom powder.

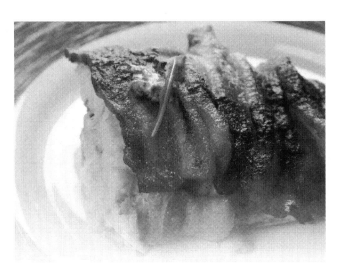

BAKED COD WRAPPED IN BACON

Preparation Time: 10 minutes
Cooking Time: 20 minutes
Servings: 2

Nutrition:
- calories 561,
- fat 9g,
- fiber 2g,
- carbs 8g,

Ingredients:
- 2 Cod fillets
- 1 tbsp. olive oil
- 4 slices bacon
- Lemon wedges
- 2 tbsp. tarragon

Directions:
1. Preheat the oven to 350°F.

2. Pat the filets dry.

3. Wrap bacon around the cod filets.

4. Place fillets on a roasting tray, and drizzle with olive oil.

5. Bake for 15-20 minutes.

6. Garnish with lemon wedges and chopped tarragon.

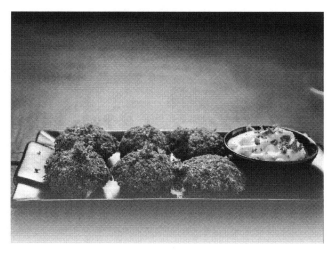

Falafel and Tahini Sauce

Preparation Time: 10 minutes
Cooking Time: 10 minutes
Servings: 2

Nutrition:
- Calories: 281,
- Fat: 24 g
- Carbohydrates: 5 g
- Protein: 8 g

Ingredients:
- ½ tablespoon ground coriander
- 1 teaspoon kosher salt
- 1 tablespoon ground cumin
- 1 cup raw cauliflower, pureed
- 2 large eggs
- 3 tablespoons coconut flour
- 1 clove garlic, minced
- ½ teaspoon cayenne pepper
- ½ cup ground slivered almonds
- 2 tablespoons fresh parsley, chopped

Tahini sauce:
- 1 tablespoon lemon juice
- 1 clove garlic, minced
- 2 tablespoons tahini paste
- 3 tablespoons water
- ½ teaspoon kosher salt, more to taste if desired

Directions:

1. For the cauliflower, you should end up with a cup of the puree. It takes about 1 medium head (florets only) to get that much. First, chop it up with a knife, then add it to a food processor or magic bullet and pulse until it's blended but still has a grainy texture.

2. You can grind the almonds in a similar manner – just don't over grind them, you want the texture.

3. Combine the ground cauliflower and ground almonds in a medium bowl. Add the rest of the ingredients and stir until well blended.

4. Heat a half and half mix of olive and grape seed (or any other light oil) oil until sizzling. While it's heating, form the mix into 8 three-inch patties that are about the thickness of a hockey puck.

5. Fry them four at a time until browned on one side and then flip and cook the other side. Resist the urge to flip too soon – you should see the edges turning brown before you attempt it – maybe 4 minutes or so per side. Remove to a plate lined with a paper towel to drain any excess oil.

6. Serve with tahini sauce, and a tomato & parsley garnish if desired.

Tahini sauce: Blend all ingredients in a bowl. Thin with more water if you like a lighter consistency.

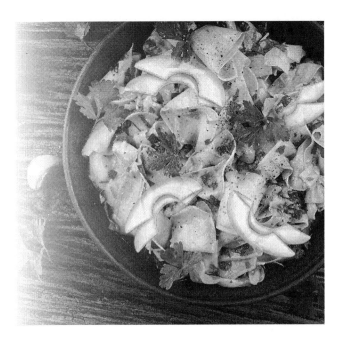

4. Set the avocado and zucchini and on a plate in an overlapping manner.
5. Now drizzle the lemon juice mixture over the salad.
6. Top the salad with the finely chopped almonds.

Zucchini Carpaccio

Preparation Time: 10 minutes
Cooking Time: 0 minute
Servings: 2

Nutrition:
- Calories: 81,
- Carbs: 5 g
- Fat: 6 g
- Protein: 3 g

Ingredients:

3 Cups thinly sliced zucchini
1 Thinly sliced ripe avocado
1 tablespoon freshly squeezed lemon juice
1 tablespoon Extra-virgin olive oil
¼ tablespoon finely grated lemon zest
½ teaspoon freshly ground black pepper
1 ounce Sliced and chopped almonds
Sea salt to taste

Directions:

1. Mix the lemon juice with the lemon zest in a bowl.
2. Add in the olive oil along with black pepper and sea salt.
3. Thinly slice the zucchini and avocado on a plate.

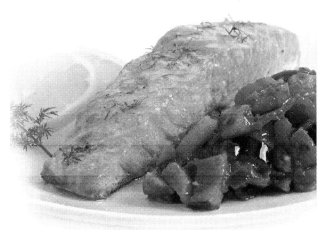

Salmon with Salsa

Preparation Time: 15 min
Cooking Time: 8 min
Servings: 2

Nutrition:
- Calories: 481,
- Fat: 37.2 g
- Carbohydrates: 15 g
- Fiber: 9.6 g
- Protein: 29.9 g

Ingredients:

For Salsa:

- 1 small tomato, chopped
- 1 eggplant cut into thin slices
- 2 tablespoons red onion, chopped finely
- ¼ cup fresh cilantro, chopped finely
- 1 tablespoon Extra-virgin
- 1 tablespoon jalapeño pepper, seeded and minced finely
- 1 garlic clove, minced finely
- Salt and ground black pepper, as required

For Salmon:
- 4 (5-ounces) (1-inch thick) salmon fillets
- 3 tablespoons butter
- 1 tablespoon fresh rosemary leaves, chopped
- 1 tablespoon fresh lemon juice

Directions:

1. For salsa: Heat a pan with extra virgin olive oil, add the vegetables and cook until the aubergines are cooked..

2. For salmon: season each salmon fillet with salt and black pepper generously. In a large skillet, melt butter over medium-high. Place the salmon fillets, skins side up and cook for about 4 minutes. Carefully change the side of each salmon fillet and cook for about 4 minutes more. Stir in the rosemary and lemon juice and remove from the heat. Divide the salsa onto serving plates evenly. To each plate with 1 salmon fillet and serve.

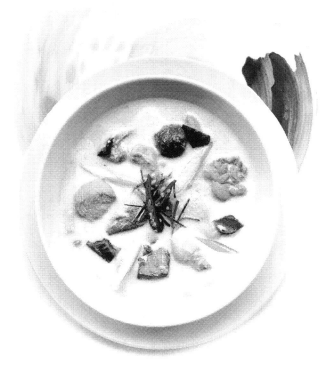

CHIPOTLE CHICKEN CHOWDER

Preparation Time: 10 minutes
Cooking Time: 25 minutes

Servings: 2
- **Nutrition:**
- Calories: 140,
- Carbs: 22 g
- Fat: 3 g
- Protein: 6 g

Ingredients:

16 ounces Boneless, skinless, fully cooked chicken breast meat

3 cups Organic chicken broth

3 cups Coconut Milk

6 tablespoons Tapioca flour

2 tablespoons Extra-virgin olive oil

2 teaspoons Ground Cumin

7 ounces chopped green bell pepper

7 ounces chopped red pepper

7 ounces chopped white onion

3 Chipotle peppers in adobo sauce

1 Cup Water

Spring onions for garnishing

Directions:

1. Over medium heat, place your thick base saucepan and add extra-virgin olive oil.

2. Add the vegetables like onion and all bell peppers along with cumin. Stir the mix thoroughly so that everything gets mixed. Cook it for a couple of minutes while stirring it occasionally.

3. Add the chicken broth, water, and chipotle.

4. Always remain careful of the quantity of chipotle you add. If you don't like it too hot, be careful with the quantity.

5. Bring the contents to a boil.

6. Reduce the heat once the mixture has come to a boil.

7. Cover the saucepan and let it simmer for good 8-10 minutes.

8. Add the chicken breasts.

9. Prepare the tapioca flour mixture in a separate bowl.
10. To make this, take the flour in a bowl and add 2/3 cup of coconut milk. Blend the mixture properly. Ensure that there are no lumps.
11. Now, add this mixture to the broth in the saucepan and let it also come to a boil.
12. Allow it boil for a few minutes and then add the remaining coconut milk to the broth.
13. Over medium heat, continue cooking the broth for a few more minutes. Keep stirring the broth at regular intervals.
14. Ensure that the soup is thick and bubbly.
15. After a few minutes, transfer the soup into a bowl and garnish with chopped green onion.

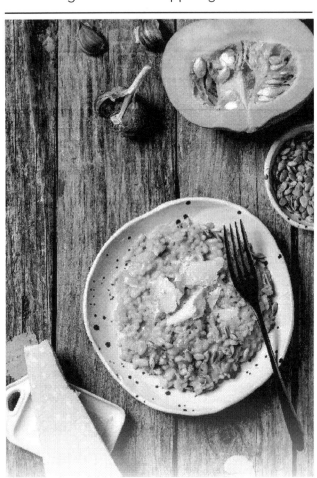

Butternut Squash Risotto

Preparation Time: 10 minutes
Cooking Time: 15 minutes
Servings: 4

Nutrition:
- Calories: 337,
- Fat: 25 g
- Carbohydrates: 9 g
- Fiber: 3 g
- Protein: 8 g

Ingredients:

Butter- 3 tablespoons
Minced sage- 2 tablespoons
Black pepper, ground up- 1/4 teaspoon
Minced rosemary- 1 teaspoon
Salt- 1 teaspoon
Dry sherry- ½ cup
Riced cauliflower- 4 cups
Butternut squash, cooked and mashed- ½ cup
Parmesan cheese, grated - ½ cup
Mascarpone cheese- ½ cup
Grated nutmeg- 1/8 teaspoon
Minced garlic- 1 teaspoon

Directions:

1. Melt your butter inside of a large frying pan turned to a medium level of heat.
2. Add your rosemary, your sage, and the garlic. Cook this for about one minute or until this mixture begins to become fragrant.
3. Add in the cauliflower rice, the pepper and salt and the mashed squash. Cook this for three minutes. You will know it is ready for the next step when cauliflower is starting to soften up for you.
4. Add in your sherry and cook this for an additional six minutes, or until the majority of the liquid is absorbed into the rice, or when the cauliflower is much softer.
5. Stir in the mascarpone cheese, the Parmesan cheese, as well as the nutmeg (grated).
6. Cook all of this on a medium heat level, being sure to stir it occasionally and do this until the

cheese has melted and the risotto has gotten creamy. This will take around four to five minutes.

7. Taste the risotto and add more pepper and salt to season if you wish.

8. Remove your pan from the burner and garnish your risotto with more of the her

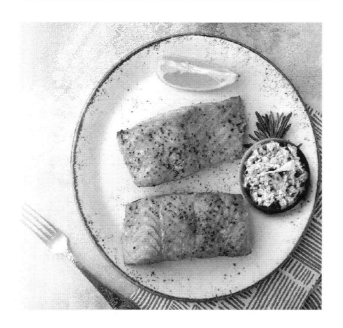

GRILLED SALMON WITH AVOCADO SALSA

Preparation Time: 15 minutes

Cooking Time: 25 minutes

Servings: 1

Nutrition:
- Calories: 232,
- Carbs: 18 g
- Fat: 5 g
- Protein: 29 g

Ingredients:
- 16 ounces Salmon
- 1 Avocado-Sliced
- ½ Red Onion-Sliced
- 1 tablespoon Olive Oil
- ½ teaspoon Paprika Powder
- ½ teaspoon Ground Cumin
- ½ teaspoon Black Pepper
- 1/4 teaspoon Chilli Powder
- Fresh Cilantro - Chopped
- 4 tablespoons Lime Juice
- Salt to taste

Directions:

1. For the seasoning mix, add the chopped onions, paprika, chilli powder, cumin, olive oil, and salt in a mixing bowl.

2. Coat the salmon properly with the prepared mix

3. Keep it in the refrigerator for at least 45 minutes

4. In a separate bowl, add the avocado, onion, cilantro, and lime juice, salt. Let it cool in the fridge for a while.

5. Grill the salmon from both sides.

6. Eat the salmon with avocado salsa on the side.

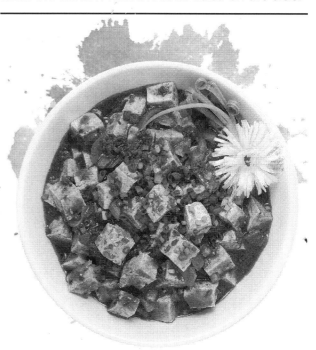

THAI TOFU CURRY

Preparation Time: 15 min

Cooking Time: 30 min

Servings: 2

Nutrition:

Calories: 146,

Carbs: 10 gr

Fat: 8 gr

Protein: 10 gr

Ingredients:

7 ounces Tofu- Small chunks

2 ounces Mangetout

2 ounces Baby corn- Cut in small pieces

1 Green chili- chopped

2 Shallots-Chopped

2 Lime leaves

1 Aubergine

½ Green pepper- thinly sliced

1/3 cup of lime juice

½ teaspoon sesame oil

1 teaspoon soy sauce

2 tablespoons green curry Thai paste

2 ounces' vegetable stock

7 ounces Coconut milk

Lime wedges for serving

6 ounces Long-grain Basmati rice for serving

Chopped coriander for garnishing

Directions:

1. Take a large skillet with deep sides.
2. Begin by frying the shallots on medium heat for about 5 minutes.
3. Add the salt as it would speed up the cooking.
4. Ensure that the shallots are translucent.
5. Toss in the chili and continue frying for another minute.
6. You'll see the color of the shallots changing. It would be time to add the curry paste.
7. Continue frying for another minute.
8. Now, add the coconut milk and the Thai sauce.
9. Let the mixture come to a boil.
10. Once the mixture has started to boil, reduce the heat and let it simmer for another 5 minutes.
11. Add the aubergine and the lime leaves. Let it cook for another 10 minutes.
12. After this, add tofu and green pepper to the curry.
13. Take off the lid and let it cook for 5 more minutes.
14. Finally, add the mange tout, baby corn, and lime juice.
15. In a separate vessel, cook your rice.
16. Sprinkle coriander on the top and put the lime wedge on the side.
17. Serve it hot with rice.

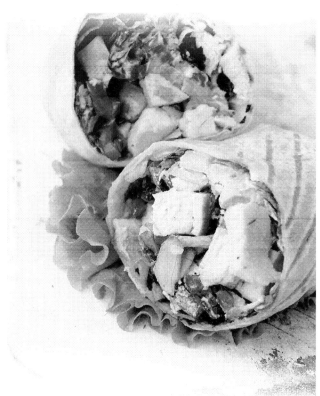

LUNCH CHICKEN WRAPS

Preparation time: 18 minutes

Cooking time: 6 hours

Servings: 6

Nutrition:
- Calories 376,
- Fat 18.5,
- Fiber 3,
- Carbs 29.43,
- Protein 23

Ingredients:

- 6 tortillas
- 3 tablespoon Caesar dressing
- 1-pound chicken breast
- ½ cup lettuce
- 1 cup water
- 1 oz. bay leaf
- 1 teaspoon salt
- 1 teaspoon ground pepper
- 1 teaspoon coriander
- 4 oz. Feta cheese

Directions:

1. Put the chicken breast in the slow cooker.
2. Sprinkle the meat with the bay leaf, salt, ground pepper, and coriander.
3. Add water and cook the chicken breast for 6 hours on LOW.
4. Then remove the cooked chicken from the slow cooker and shred it with a fork.
5. Chop the lettuce roughly.
6. Then chop Feta cheese. Combine the chopped Ingredients: together and add the shredded chicken breast and Caesar dressing.
7. Mix everything together well. After this, spread the tortillas with the shredded chicken mixture and wrap them. Enjoy!

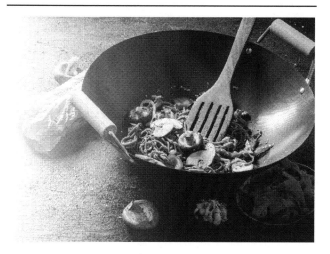

Spring Ramen Bowl

Preparation time: 15 min
Cooking time: 20 min

Servings: 4

Nutrition:
- calories 300,
- fat 12 g,
- fiber 1g,
- carbs 3g,
- protein 9g

Ingredients

3,5 oz. (100g) soba noodles

4 eggs

1 medium zucchini, julienned or grated

4 cups chicken stock

2 cups watercress

½ cup snap peas

1 cup mushrooms, finely sliced

1 leek (white part only), finely sliced

2 cloves garlic, minced

1 long red chili, seeded and finely chopped

1.6-inch ginger, minced

1 tsp. sesame oil

2 nori sheets, crumbled

1 lemon, cut into wedges

1 tbsp. olive oil

Directions

1. To boil the eggs, fill a saucepan with enough water to cover the eggs and set over medium heat. Bring water to a gentle boil. Add the eggs and cook for 7 minutes. Drain and transfer the eggs into cold water. Set aside.
2. Place a medium-sized saucepan over medium-low heat. Heat the olive oil and sauté the garlic, ginger, leek, and chili for 5 minutes. Add the stock, noodles, and sesame oil. Cook for another 8 minutes or until noodles are cooked according to your desired doneness. During the last minute, add the zucchini, mushroom, and watercress.
3. Divide the ramen between four bowls and top with nori. Serve with the eggs and lemon wedges.

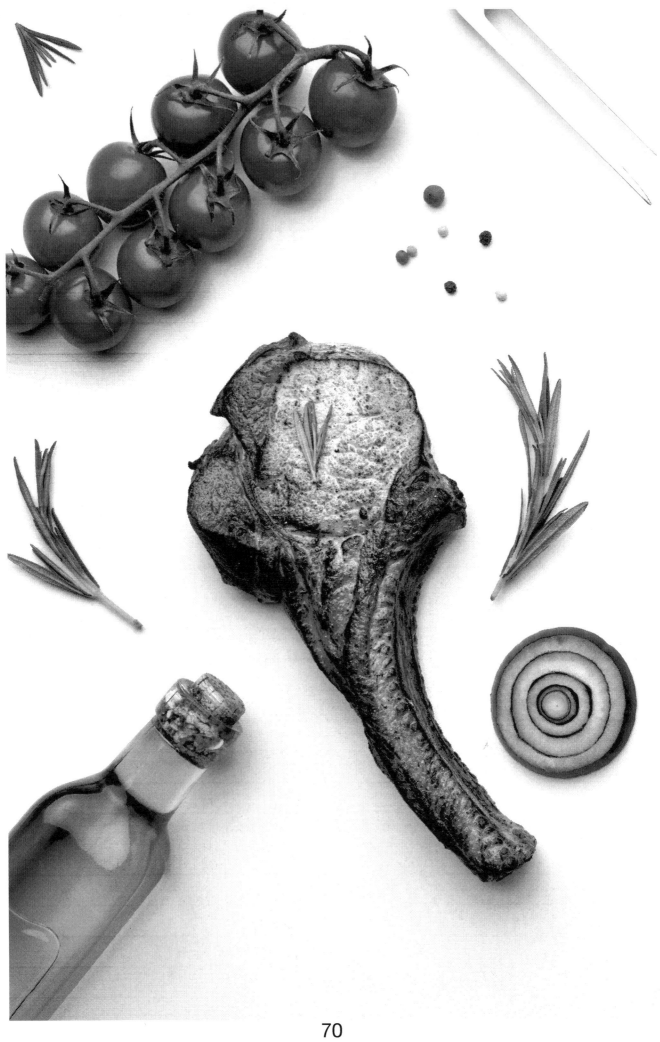

DINNER MEALS AFTER THE FAST

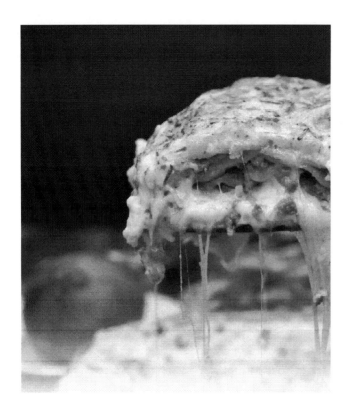

INCREDIBLY DELICIOUS LASAGNA

Preparation Time: 10 minutes
Cooking Time: 1 hour 30 minutes
Servings: 4

Nutrition:
- calories 712,
- fat 31g,
- fiber 6g,
- carbs 50g,
- protein 44g

Ingredients:

1 pound of lean grass-fed ground beef
1 (16-ounce) package of lasagna noodles
1 cup of shredded mozzarella cheese
1 onion, finely chopped
½ cup of mushrooms, finely chopped
1 pint of ricotta cheese
¼ cup of parmesan cheese, finely grated
2 eggs
1 (28-ounce) jar of spaghetti sauce
1 (16-ounce) package of cottage cheese

Direction

1. Preheat your oven to 350 degrees Fahrenheit.
2. In a large skillet over medium-high heat, add the ground beef and cook until brown.
3. Add the chopped mushrooms and onions. Cook until the mushrooms and onions have softened, stirring occasionally.
4. Stir in the spaghetti sauce and allow to heat through.
5. In a medium bowl, add the cottage cheese, ricotta cheese, and parmesan grated cheese, and eggs. Stir until well combined.
6. Spread a layer of the meat mixture to a greased baking dish.
7. Layer with lasagna noodles.
8. Spread the cheese mixture over the lasagna noodles and sprinkle with the mozzarella cheese.
9. Add another layer of meat mixture and repeat with all the ingredients. Make sure you have ½ cup of shredded mozzarella cheese left.
10. Cover the baking dish with foil and place inside your oven. Bake for 45 minutes.
11. Remove the aluminum foil and sprinkle with the remaining ½ cup of shredded mozzarella cheese. Bake for 15 minutes.
12. Remove from your oven and allow to cool. Serve and enjoy!

BEEF STROGANOFF

Preparation Time: 10 minutes
Cooking Time: 30 minutes
Servings: 6

Nutrition:
- calories 497,
- fat 22g,
- fiber 2g,

- carbs 19g,
- protein 49g

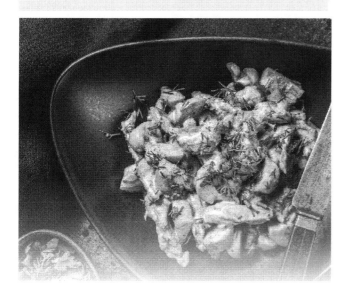

Ingredients:

- 1 (10-ounce) package of egg noodles, cooked according to the package Direction
- 2 pounds of beef steak, sliced into thin strips
- 4 tablespoons of butter
- 2 cups of brown or cremini mushrooms, sliced
- 1 large white or yellow onion, sliced
- 2 medium garlic cloves, minced
- ½ cup of sour cream
- ¼ cup of flour
- 2 teaspoons of Worcestershire sauce
- 1 teaspoon of Dijon mustard
- 1 teaspoon of smoked paprika or regular paprika
- 3 cups of homemade low-sodium beef stock
- ½ teaspoon of fine sea salt
- ½ teaspoon of freshly cracked black pepper

Direction

1. In a large skillet over medium-high heat, add 2 tablespoons of butter.
2. Add the beef strips and cook until brown. Remove and set aside.
3. Add the remaining 2 tablespoons of butter to the skillet along with the sliced mushrooms, chopped onion and minced garlic. Sauté until vegetables have softened, stirring occasionally.
4. Sprinkle ¼ cup of flour over the vegetables and cook for another minute, stirring occasionally.
5. Lower the heat and stir in the beef stock while whisking constantly. Allow to simmer until thickens.
6. Stir in the Worcestershire sauce, Dijon mustard, smoked paprika and sour cream until well combined.
7. Stir in the beef strips and simmer for another 5 minutes.
8. Serve over egg noodles.

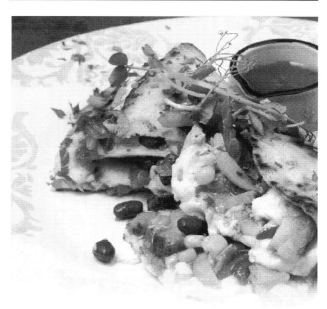

NO CHEESE QUESADILLAS

Preparation Time: 10 min
Cooking Time: 30 min
Servings: 3

Nutrition:

- calories 191,
- fat 9g,
- fiber 2g,
- carbs 8g,
- protein 20g

Ingredients:

Extra chunky salsa, as required

12 yellow no oil corn tortillas

2 medium onions, chopped

1 small yellow bell pepper, chopped

1 small green bell pepper, chopped

1 small red bell pepper, chopped

1 ½ cups no oil refried pinto beans

1 ½ cups baby corn

Chilli powder, to taste

Direction:

1. Place a tortilla on your countertop. Spread 4 tbsp refried beans and corn over it.
2. Sprinkle a little of onions, bell peppers and chilli powder over it.
3. Cover with another tortilla.
4. Place a nonstick pan over medium heat. Carefully lift the quesadilla and place on the pan. Cook until the underside is crisp. Flip sides and cook the other side until crisp.
5. Repeat steps 1-4 to make remaining quesadillas.
6. Cut each into 4 wedges and serve with salsa.

Kamut Savory Salad

Preparation Time: 10 min

Cooking Time: 20 min

Servings: 5

Nutrition:
- calories 170,
- fat 8g,
- fiber 2g,
- carbs 8g,
- protein 4g

Ingredients:

1 cup kamut grain, soaked in water overnight, drained

¼ cup frozen mixed vegetables

1 small carrot, chopped

½ cup mixed bell pepper, chopped

1 small onion, chopped

¼ cup canned or cooked red kidney beans

1 tsp olive oil

3 cups vegetable stock

Salt to taste

Pepper to taste

Spring onion, to garnish

Parsley, to garnish

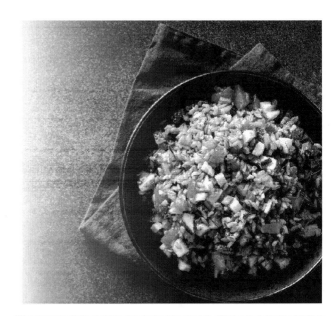

Direction:

1. Add kamut and stock into a saucepan. Place a saucepan over medium heat. Cook until tender. Set aside.
2. Place a pan over medium heat. Add oil. When the oil is heated, add onion and sauté until translucent.
3. Add rest of the ingredients and stir. Heat thoroughly.
4. Sprinkle spring onions and parsley and serve.

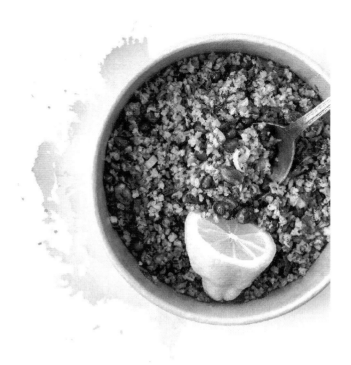

Freekeh Salad

Preparation Time: 10 minutes
Cooking Time: 10 minutes
Servings: 2

Nutrition:
- calories 800,
- fat 8g,
- fiber 2g,
- carbs 12g,
- protein 69g

Ingredients:

2 vine tomatoes, chopped or 4 cherry tomatoes, quartered

Sea salt to taste

2 tbsp olive oil

Juice of ½ lemon

Zest of ½ lemon, grated

A handful fresh cilantro or parsley, chopped

1 small cucumber, chopped

½ cup corn kernels

1 small onion, chopped

¾ cup freekeh

2 cups water

To serve:

Hummus or pesto as required

Avocado slices

Mini tortillas or wraps, as required

Direction:

1. Add freekeh and water. Place water over medium heat. When it begins to boil, lower the heat and cover with a lid. Simmer for 10-12 minutes. Uncover and cook until tender. Drain and set aside.

2. Add lemon juice, oil, zest, salt and pepper into a small bowl and whisk well.

3. Add rest of the ingredients including freekeh into a bowl and toss well. Pour dressing on top and toss well. Chill until ready to use.

4. Spread tortillas on your countertop. Place salad on one half of the tortillas. Top with avocado and hummus. Fold the other half over the filling and serve.

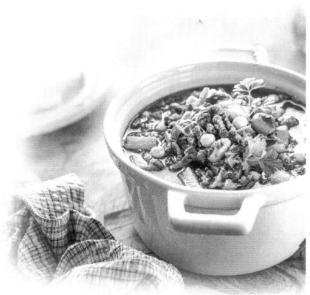

Kamut, Lentil, and Chickpea Soup

Preparation Time: 10 minutes
Cooking Time: 50 minutes
Servings: 9

Nutrition:
- calories 800,
- fat 8g,
- fiber 2g,
- carbs 12g,
- protein 69g

Ingredients:

1 ½ cups kamut berries, rinsed

4 tbsp olive oil

2 cups carrots, finely chopped

1 cup celery, thinly sliced

4 tsp fresh thyme, chopped

4 cloves garlic, minced

4 bay leaves

½ tsp pepper powder

A handful celery leaves, chopped (optional)

4 cups boiling water

4 cups onion, finely chopped

1 ½ cups fresh parsley, chopped

2 tbsp chopped fresh thyme

8 cans (14.5 ounces each) chicken broth or use equivalent homemade broth

2/3 cup dried lentils, rinsed, soaked in water for 20 minutes

2 cans (15 ounces each) chickpeas, rinsed, drained

Direction:

1. Add kamut into a bowl. Cover with boiling water. Let it soak for 30 minutes.
2. Place a soup pot over medium heat. Add oil. When the oil is heated, add onion and herbs and sauté until onions are translucent.
3. Add garlic and sauté until fragrant.
4. Add rest of the ingredients except chickpeas and stir. Cover and cook until tender.
5. Ladle into soup bowls. Sprinkle celery and serve.

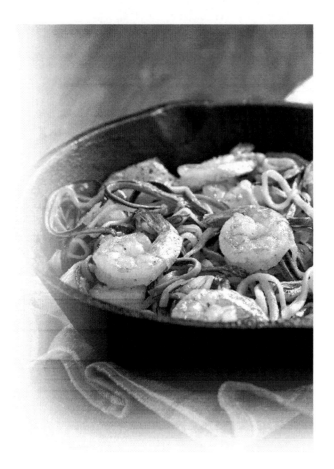

Garlic Shrimp with Zucchini Noodles

Preparation Time: 10 minutes

Cooking Time: 4 minutes

Servings: 3

Nutrition:
- calories 280,
- fat 8g,
- fiber 3g,
- carbs 8g,
- protein 6g

Ingredients

1 lb. shrimp, shelled and deveined

2 medium zucchinis, spiraled

2 tbsps. Fresh chives, minced

2 tbsps. Fresh lemon juice

4 garlic cloves, minced

2 tbsps. Coconut oil

Sea salt

Freshly ground black pepper

Directions

1. Place a skillet over medium heat and heat the oil.
2. Sauté the garlic about 2-3 minutes.
3. Add the shrimp and cook 2-4 minutes or until pink. Remove the shrimp from the pan.
4. Add the lemon juice and stir. Bring the mixture to a boil and simmer until most of the liquid has evaporated.
5. Mix in the zucchini noodles and continue to cook another 3-4 minutes.
6. Bring the shrimp back to the skillet and season to taste. Stir well and sprinkle with chives before serving.

Filipino Chicken Adobo

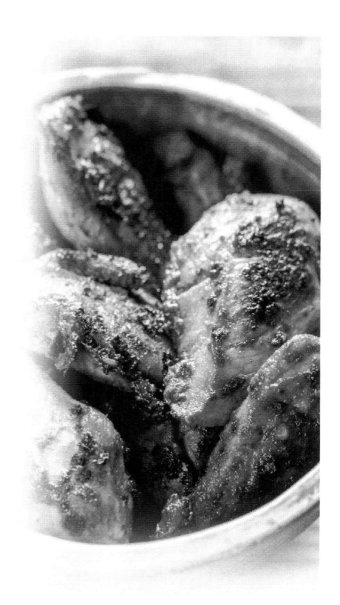

Preparation Time: 10 minutes
Cooking Time: 20 minutes
Servings: 4
Nutrition:

- calories 207,
- fat 8g,
- fiber 2g,
- carbs 8g,
- protein 6g

Ingredients

- 1 lb. boneless chicken, cut into pieces
- 2 tbsps. Soy sauce
- 3 tbsps. Apple cider vinegar
- 1½ tsps. Garlic, minced
- 2 tbsps. Olive oil

Directions

1. Mix the soy sauce, vinegar, garlic, and oil in a pan.
2. Add the chicken and coat it with the soy sauce mixture.
3. Place the pan over medium heat, add the chicken, cover with a lid, and let it simmer 10-15 minutes.
4. Uncover the pan and adjust the heat to medium-high. Cook until the chicken is browned. Stir occasionally to avoid burning.
5. Serve and enjoy!

Quick and Easy Squash Soup

Preparation Time: 5 minutes
Cooking Time: 15 minutes
Servings: 1

Nutrition:
- calories 108,
- fat 8g,
- fiber 2g,
- carbs 8g,
- protein 7g

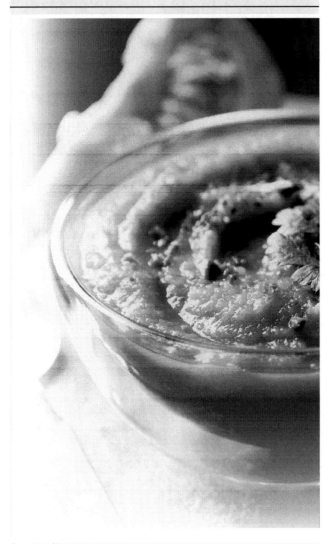

Ingredients

1 tbsp of olive oil

1 cup of chopped onions

1 cup of chopped squash

2 cups of chicken broth

1 tbsp of Greek yogurt

½ tsp of nutmeg

½ tsp of salt

1 tsp of pepper

Direction

1. Deposit your 1 tablespoon of olive oil into a large saucepan, before adding your 1 cup of chopped onions, your 1 cup of chopped squash, your 2 cups of chicken broth, your ½ teaspoon of nutmeg, your ¼ teaspoon of salt, and your 1 teaspoon of pepper.

2. Stir everything together well and cook for 15 minutes under high heat.

3. To serve, add a tbsp of yogurt.

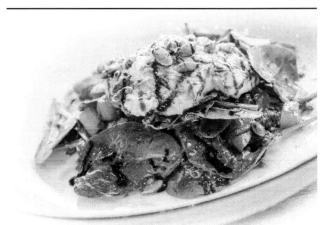

Sesame-Ginger Chicken Salad

Preparation Time: 10 min

Cooking Time: 10 min

Servings: 2

Nutrition:
- calories 340,
- fat 8g,
- fiber 2g,
- carbs 8g,
- protein 6g

Ingredients

3 oz. cooked chicken breast, shredded

4 cups romaine lettuce, chopped

¼ cup carrot, shredded

½ cup fresh spinach

¼ cup radishes, sliced

1 scallion, sliced

3 tablespoons Sugar-free sesame-ginger dressing

Direction

1. In a medium-sized salad bowl, mix all the ingredients (except for the sesame-ginger dressing) and toss well.
2. Add the dressing and toss well. Serve and enjoy!

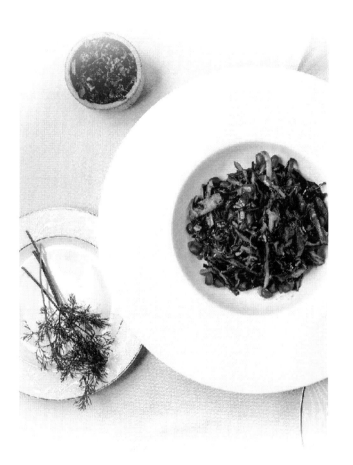

REDS SALAD ON BACON AND BALSAMIC VINAIGRETTE

Preparation Time: 10 minutes
Cooking Time: 30 minutes
Servings: 3

Nutrition:
- calories 108,
- fat 50g,
- fiber 2g,
- carbs 8g,
- protein 48g

Ingredients

1 head red leaf lettuce, torn
2 red oak leaf lettuce, torn
½ cup radicchio, julienned
6 streaky bacon
2 tablespoons extra virgin olive oil
1/8 cup balsamic vinegar
2 garlic cloves, grated
1 tablespoon Dijon mustard
Dash of red pepper flakes
Pinch of sea salt, add more if needed
Pinch of black pepper, add more if needed

Direction

1. For the dressing, pour olive oil into a nonstick skillet. Fry streaky bacon for 3 minutes or until golden brown. Transfer to a plate and crumble into small pieces. Set aside
2. In the same pan, add in garlic, balsamic vinegar, Dijon mustard, red pepper flakes, salt, and pepper. Whisk until mixture is well blended. Set aside
3. To assemble, in a big salad bowl, put together red leaf lettuce, red oak leaf lettuce, and radicchio. Drizzle in dressing. Top with bacon bits. Serve.

VEGGIE-STUFFED OMELET

Preparation Time: 10 minutes
Cooking Time: 30 minutes
Servings: 1

Nutrition:
- calories 150,
- fat 8g,
- fiber 2g,
- carbs 8g,
- protein 24g

Ingredients

2 eggs, beaten

¼ cup mushrooms, sliced

1 cup loosely packed contemporary baby spinach leaves, rinsed

2 tablespoons Red bell pepper, chopped

1 tablespoon onion, chopped

1 tablespoon reduced-fat cheddar cheese, shredded

1 teaspoon olive or canola oil

1 tablespoon water

Dash salt

Dash pepper

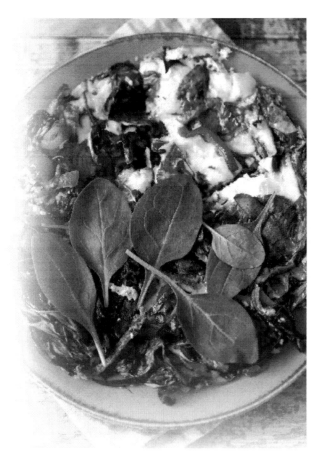

Direction

1. Heat oil in an 8-inch nonstick skillet. Sauté the mushrooms, onion, and bell pepper for about 2 minutes until the onion is tender. Add the spinach and continue to cook, stirring frequently, until the spinach wilts. Once cooked, transfer the vegetables to a small bowl.

2. In a medium bowl, whisk the beaten eggs, water, salt, and pepper until well combined.

3. Place the same skillet in which you cooked the vegetable mixture over medium-high heat. Add the egg mixture immediately. Make a quick, sliding back-and-forth motion with the pan, using a spatula to spread the eggs at the bottom of the pan. Once the mixture is applied, let it stand for a few seconds to brown the bottom of the omelet lightly. Do not overcook it.

4. Carefully place the vegetable mixture on the half side of the omelet. Top it with cheese and, using a spatula, gently fold the other half over the vegetables. Transfer the veggie-stuffed omelet to a plate and serve.

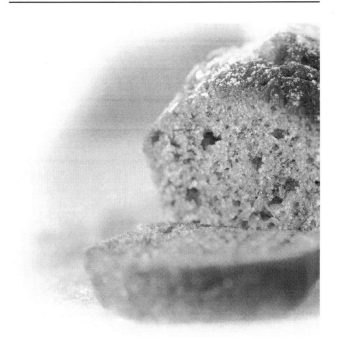

COCONUT BANANA BREAD

Preparation Time: 10 min

Cooking Time: 55 min

Servings: 6

Nutrition:
- calories 223,
- fat 8g,
- fiber 2g,
- carbs 8g,
- protein 3g

Ingredients

Small bananas 3 ripe

Syrup of Rice malt 90 g

Lightly whisked eggs 3 medium

Bicarbonate of Soda, three fourth teaspoon

Vanilla extract which is alcohol free, a few drop

Salt, half teaspoon

Coconut flour 30 g

For serving, Fruit

Direction

1. Settle the oven to 180 ° C and do the greasing of a tin of twenty-one into nine cm. bars.
2. Please take off the peel of bananas and make a puree of them in a small bowl. Then put the eggs, vanilla, rice malt syrup, and combine.
3. Add bicarbonate soda, flour, and salt and whisk well. In a prepared tin, put the mixture.
4. Then keep it for baking for 50 minutes or until the spatula in the center of the bread can come out clear. Cool entirely on a wire rack in a tin, then make a slice and present with fruit.

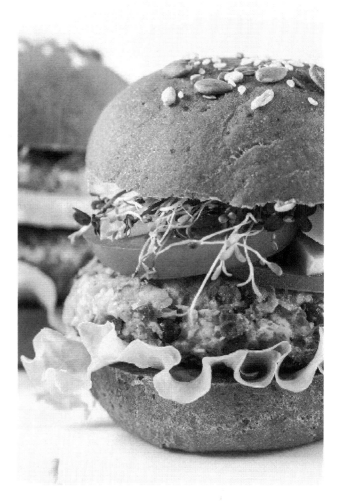

VEGAN LENTIL BURGER

Preparation Time: 10 minutes

Cooking Time: 2 hours

Servings: 6

Nutrition:
- calories 560,
- fat 14g,
- fiber 2g,
- carbs 65g,
- protein 21g

Ingredients
- Brown lentils 3/4 cup
- Extra-virgin olive oil 2 teaspoons
- Low-sodium vegetable broth or water 1 and 3/4 cups
- Red onion, half thinly sliced and half chopped 1 large
- Juice of half lemon
- Kosher salt
- Fresh spinach 8 ounces
- Garlic cloves, minced 2 large
- Black pepper
- Ground cumin, half teaspoon
- Whole-wheat bread crumbs 1 cup
- Cooking spray
- Walnuts, toasted and finely chopped half cup
- Whole-grain vegan buns 6

Direction

1. Take the lentils and 1 3/4 cup of the broth for boiling on high temperature in a medium saucepan. Decrease heat to medium-low, partly covered, and cook until the lentils are entirely

softened. The liquid is absorbed for around 30 minutes.

2. Mix it with the leftover one tablespoon of the broth and mix well with the stick blender. Set it aside.

3. Warm the oil over the medium temperature in a large nonstick skillet. Add the lemon juice, chopped onion, and 1/4 teaspoon salt and cook for around 6 minutes, stirring till soft.

4. Add the spinach, garlic, 1 and a half teaspoons of black pepper and cumin, and stir until the spinach is withered for around 3 minutes.

1. Add the mixture of spinach, breadcrumbs, walnuts, and salt to the lentils and blend thoroughly. Put a cover and refrigerate for at least one hour or overnight.

2. Heat the grill to medium-high. Shape the mixture into six 4-inch patties and sprinkle each side with a cooking spray. Grill till pleasant grill marks is formed, around 3 minutes per hand. Put the patties in the buns with the chopped onion and other seasonings and eat.

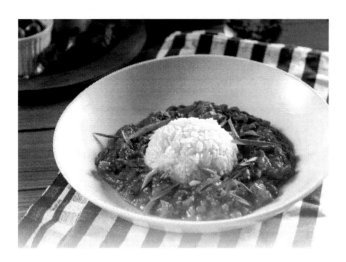

Picadillo Chicken

Preparation Time: 10 minutes
Cooking Time: 40 minutes
Servings: 6

Nutrition:
- calories 200,
- fat 8g,
- fiber 2g,
- carbs 8g,
- protein 24g

Ingredients:

2 tbsp oil

1 tsp ground cumin

2/3 cup chicken broth

1 pound lean ground beef

3 cup red beans, precooked

2 cup tomato sauce

Salt and pepper to taste

1/2 white onion, diced small

2 garlic cloves, minced

3 large carrots, peeled and diced small

Direction

1. In a preheated Dutch oven, add oil, onions, and garlic, and sauté until translucent.

2. Add the ground beef, carrots, and beans.

3. Pour in the tomato sauce and chicken broth. Then add the cumin, salt, and pepper; mix well.

4. Cook for 40 minutes or until the meat and carrots are cooked through and tender.

5. Delicious served on rice.

Instant Pot Teriyaki Chicken

Preparation Time: 10 minutes
Cooking Time: 20 minutes
Servings: 6

Nutrition:
- calories 200,
- fat 8g,

- fiber 2g,
- carbs 8g,
- protein 6g
- calories 200,

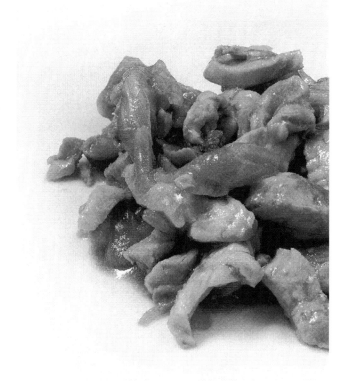

Ingredients:

¼ c. soy sauce or Bragg's Liquid Aminos

1 ½ tsp. ginger paste

1 c. water

1/3 c. honey

2 cloves of garlic, minced

2 pounds chicken breasts, cut into strips

2 med. green onions, sliced

3 tbsp. rice wine vinegar

For slurry:

¼ c. cold water

2 tbsp of extra virgin olive oil

3 tbsp. cornstarch

Direction

1. Heat the oil in a deep pan and fry the chicken for a few minutes.
2. Add the water, honey, soy sauce, vinegar, garlic, and ginger. Stir to incorporate, then lay the chicken breasts on top of the liquid.
3. Cook covered for 10 minutes.
4. Mix the slurry in a small bowl, making sure there are no starch lumps, then pour it over the chicken.
5. Stir the chicken to incorporate the slurry, as this will thicken the sauce. Cook for a few more minutes, occasionally stirring until the sauce has reached the desired thickness.
6. Serve over rice, salads, quinoa, or whatever you prefer!

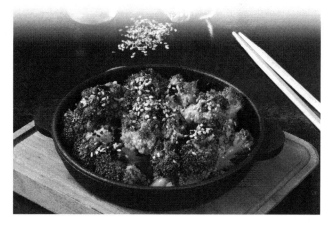

ROASTED BROCCOLI WITH LEMON

Preparation Time: 10 min

Cooking Time: 40 min

Servings: 2

Nutrition:
- calories 172
- fat 8g,
- fiber 2g,
- carbs 8g,
- protein 6g

Ingredients

Broccoli 1 large head (one and half pounds), cut into stems and florets

Freshly ground pepper

Kosher salt

Minced shallot 1 teaspoon

Olive oil (extra-virgin) 1/4 cup

Fresh lemon juice 2 teaspoons

Pine nuts 1 1/2 tablespoons

Direction

1. Settle the oven to 400 ° C. Place the broccoli flowers and stems on a wide baking sheet with two tbsp. of olive oil and sprinkle with salt.

2. Bake the broccoli in the oven for around 30 minutes, stirring halfway through, till tender and browned.

3. Meanwhile, in a small pan, roast the pine nuts on moderate flame unless golden for approximately four minutes.

4. In a small pan, combine the lemon juice with a shallot and the leftover 2 tablespoons of olive oil; sprinkle with salt and pepper. Spread the broccoli in a serving dish. Then put the toasted nuts of pine and dressing, garnish well and present.

Chicken Tetrazzini

Preparation Time: 15 minutes

Cooking Time: 25 minutes

Servings: 7

Nutrition:
- calories 163,
- fat 8g,
- fiber 2g,
- carbs 8g,
- protein 11g

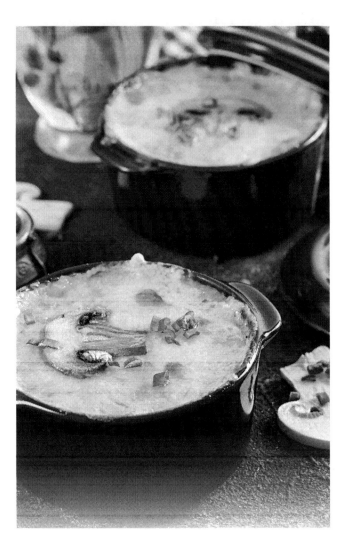

Ingredients:

¼ c. parmesan cheese, grated

1 c. mozzarella cheese, shredded

1 lb. chicken breast, boneless, skinless, & cubed

1 lb. whole wheat spaghetti noodles

1 med. onion, diced

1 tsp. oregano, dried

10 oz. button mushrooms, sliced

2 c. milk

2 med. bell peppers, diced

2 tbsp. extra virgin olive oil

3 c. chicken broth

3 lg. stalks celery, diced

3 tbsp. breadcrumbs

Sea salt & pepper, to taste

Direction

1. Warm a large pot or Dutch oven over medium heat and warm the oil in it.

2. Combine celery and onion into the pot, stirring completely to combine and allowing to cook for about three minutes or until shiny.

3. Stir the salt, pepper, mushrooms, peppers, and oregano into the pot and stir occasionally until all ingredients get shiny and begin to cook through.

4. Stir broth, milk, parmesan cheese, and chicken into the pot and stir until completely combined.

5. Break pasta noodles in half and stir them into the mixture, doing your best to get them spread evenly throughout the pot.

6. Cover and allow to cook for about ten minutes.

7. In a medium mixing bowl, combine mozzarella and breadcrumbs, mixing completely.

8. Uncover the pot and stir once more before sprinkling the cheese and crumb mixture on top. Cover and let cook for about three to five more minutes, or until the cheese is nice and bubbly.

9. Serve hot!

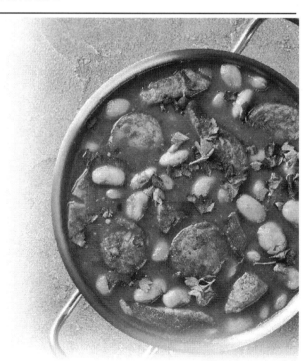

MEXICAN PORK STEW

Preparation Time: 10 minutes
Cooking Time: 45 minutes
Servings: 8

Nutrition:
- calories 291,
- fat 8g,
- fiber 8g,
- carbs 21g,
- protein 11g

Ingredients:

1 tablespoon of extra-virgin olive oil

1 pound of pork shoulder, cut into bite-sized pieces

8-ounces of sausage, cut into bite-sized pieces

1 (28-ounce) can of diced tomatoes

1 (28-ounce) can of white kidney beans, drained and rinsed

2 cups of homemade low-sodium beef stock

1 medium white or yellow onion, finely chopped

3 medium garlic cloves, minced

1 jalapeno pepper, finely chopped

1 tablespoon of smoked paprika

1 tablespoon of mild chili powder

1 teaspoon of ground cumin

½ teaspoon of fine sea salt

½ teaspoon of freshly cracked black pepper

¼ teaspoon of cayenne pepper

¼ cup of fresh cilantro, finely chopped

Direction

1. In a large Dutch oven over medium-high heat, add the extra-virgin olive oil.

2. Once hot, add the pork pieces and sausage pieces. Cook for 6 to 8 minutes, stirring occasionally

3. Add the chopped onion, minced garlic and chopped jalapeno.

4. Add all the seasonings and diced tomatoes, beans and beef stock. Give a good stir before covering with a lid. Allow to cook for 25 minutes.

5. Garnish with fresh cilantro.

6. Serve and enjoy!

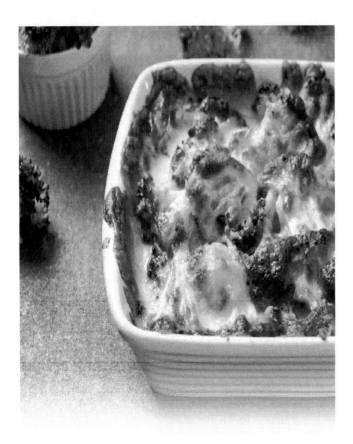

Ham and Broccoli Casserole

Preparation Time: 10 minutes

Cooking Time: 50 minutes

Servings: 8

Nutrition:
- calories 321,
- fat 8g,
- fiber 3g,
- carbs 8g,
- protein 22g

Ingredients:

2 pounds of broccoli florets

3 tablespoons of extra-virgin olive oil or other cooking fat

1 teaspoon of fine sea salt

1 teaspoon of freshly cracked black pepper

10 ounces of ham steak, cut into cubes

½ cup of heavy cream

¼ cup of homemade low-sodium chicken stock

2 cups of cheddar cheese, shredded

1 cup of mozzarella cheese, shredded

4-ounces of cream cheese, softened and cubed

2 medium garlic cloves, minced

Direction

1. Preheat your oven to 400 degrees Fahrenheit.
2. In a large casserole dish, evenly spread the broccoli florets and drizzle with the extra-virgin olive oil. Sprinkle with fine sea salt and freshly cracked black pepper.
3. Place inside your oven and bake for 15 to 20 minutes.
4. In a saucepan over medium-low heat, add the heavy cream, chicken stock, all the cheeses except for 1 cup of cheddar cheese and minced garlic. Cook until the broccoli is done, stirring constantly.
5. Remove the casserole dish from your oven and top with the ham. Pour the cheese mixture over the casserole and sprinkle with the remaining 1 cup of cheddar cheese.
6. Return to your oven and bake for another 15 minutes.
7. Carefully remove from your oven and allow to cool.
8. Serve and enjoy!

Mixed Vegetables and Chicken Egg Rolls

Preparation Time: 10 minutes

Cooking Time: 15 minutes

Servings: 4

Nutrition:
- calories 260,
- fat 8g,
- fiber 1g,
- carbs 8g,

- protein 23g

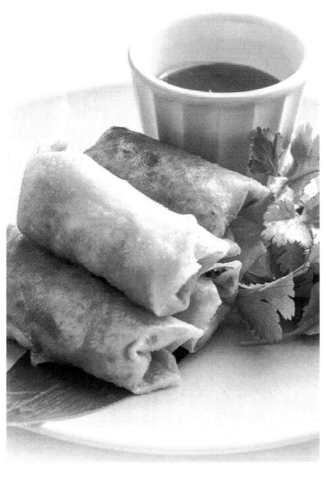

Ingredients

1 tablespoon garlic, grated

1 tablespoon ginger, grated

4 tablespoons palm sugar, crumbled

1 banana chili, minced

4 tablespoons fish sauce

Pinch of black pepper

4 tablespoons of rice wine vinegar

1 bird eye chili, minced

8 pieces spring roll wrappers

Olive oil

Water, for sealing

1 garlic clove, minced

1 shallot, julienned

¼ cup chicken, cooked shredded

1 cup bean sprouts

1 tablespoon chicken concentrate

2 tablespoons coconut oil

¼ cup squash, julienned

¼ cup carrots, julienned

¼ cup sweet potato, julienned

¼ cup potato, julienned

½ cup of water

Pinch of sea salt

Pinch of black pepper

Direction

1. Combine dipping sauce ingredients in a bowl. Stir until sugar dissolves. Taste; adjust seasoning if needed. Set aside.

2. To make spring rolls: pour coconut oil into large wok set over medium heat. Sauté garlic and shallot until limp and transparent; except for bean sprouts, add in remaining filling ingredients. Cook until root crops are fork tender. Toss in bean sprouts; stir. Turn off the heat immediately. Allow filling to cool completely to room temperature before rolling.

3. Add an equal portion of vegetable filling into spring roll paper; roll tightly, tucking in the edges and sealing with water. Set aside. Repeat step for remaining filling/wrapper.

4. Half-fill deep fryer with cooking oil set at medium heat; wait for the oil to become slightly rolls. Cook only until spring rolls turn golden brown, about 7 minutes. Transfer cooked pieces on a plate lined with paper towels. Place 2 spring rolls on a plate; serve with dipping sauce on the side.

CAULIFLOWER MASHED POTATOES

Preparation Time: 10 minutes

Cooking Time: 22 minutes

Servings: 3

Nutrition:
- calories 104,
- fat 8g,
- fiber 2g,
- carbs 8g,
- protein 2.5g

Ingredients

1 cup of chopped cauliflower

2 tablespoons of heavy cream

2 tablespoons of melted butter

1 tablespoon of mayonnaise

½ teaspoon of salt

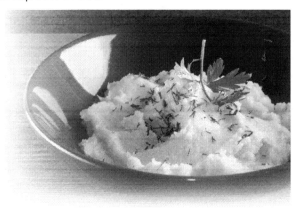

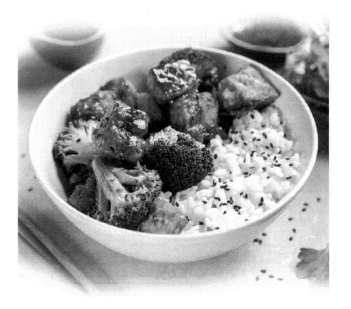

Direction

1. Set your oven to 3750 F.
2. While your oven is heating up, place your 1 cup of chopped cauliflower into a heat resistant bowl followed by your 2 tablespoons of water, drizzled over the surface of the cauliflower just to make sure that maintain moisture.
3. Cook in the microwave for about 3 minutes.
4. Now take out of the microwave, deposit cauliflower into a blender, followed by your 1 tablespoon of mayonnaise, and your ½ teaspoon of salt.
5. Blend for about 1 minute before pouring the blended ingredients into your casserole dish.
6. Drizzle your 2 tablespoons of melted butter on top and stick the dish into the oven
7. Cook for 15 minutes.
8. Serve when ready.

GINGER ORANGE STIR-FRY WITH TOFU

Preparation Time: 10 minutes

Cooking Time: 30 minutes

Servings: 4

Nutrition:
- calories 443,
- fat 8g,
- fiber 1g,
- carbs 8g,
- protein 3g

Ingredients

1 medium bunch of broccolis, cut into florets

1 block of organic extra-firm tofu, cut into 1/2 – inch cubes

1 tablespoon fresh ginger, grated

2 cloves of garlic

¼ cup of coconut sugar

2 tablespoons Tamari

1 tablespoon of rice wine vinegar

½ cup of water

1 tablespoon arrowroot starch

1 cup of frozen edamame

2 tablespoons Unrefined coconut oil

½ cup of raw cashews

2 green onions, chopped

1 tablespoon of sesame seeds

1 cup of fresh orange juice

4 servings of cooked brown rice

Direction

1. Place fruit juice in a very tiny pan over medium heat. Add the garlic, ginger, tamari, coconut sugar, and vinegar. Mix well and maintain heat until it simmers. Reduce heat to low to take care of a delicate simmer. Continue to cook another 10 minutes.

2. Set a large saucepan over medium-high heat and heat coconut oil. Sauté tofu for 5 minutes until slightly browned.

3. Add the edamame and broccoli. Continue to sauté another 5 minutes or until the broccoli is tender.

4. Dissolve arrowroot starch in water. Add it to the ginger-orange sauce and adjust heat to medium while whisking continuously. Cook another minute or until the consistency thickens. Remove pan from the heat.

5. Pour the sauce over the tofu and vegetables. Add the cashews and mix well. Remove pan from heat.

6. To serve, pour over brown rice. Top with green onions and sesame seeds.

Turkey Breast in Tomato Sauce

Preparation Time: 10 min

Cooking Time: 10 min

Servings: 2

Nutrition:
- calories 100,
- fat 8g,
- fiber 2g,
- carbs 8g,
- protein 2.5g

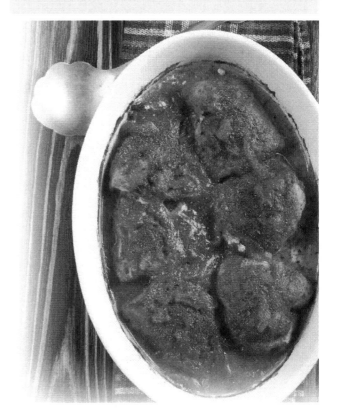

Ingredients

1 cup turkey breast, boneless, skinless cubed

¾ cup tomato sauce

½ teaspoon hot pepper sauce

1 teaspoon extra virgin olive oil

½ teaspoon ground cloves

½ cup onion, chopped finely

¼ teaspoon mustard powder

Pinch of pepper

2 cups spinach, cooked

Direction

1. Heat olive oil in a saucepan set over medium heat. Sauté onion for 3 minutes or until the onion starts to soften.

2. Add in mustard, tomato sauce, hot pepper sauce, ground cloves, and pepper. Reduce heat. Allow simmering for 5 minutes.

3. To serve, divide cooked spinach between plates. Pour cooked marinated turkey breast.

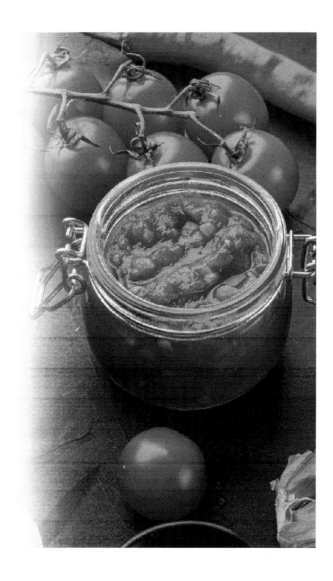

1 teaspoon of cilantro

1 tablespoon of lime juice

¼ teaspoon of kosher salt

Direction

1. Get out a blender and add your ½ cup of chopped onion, your 1 tablespoon of chopped garlic, your ¼ cup of chopped jalapeño, a ½ cup of chopped tomatoes, your 1 teaspoon of cilantro, your 1 tablespoon of lime juice, and your ¼ teaspoon of kosher salt.

2. Now pulse ingredients in the blender 4 or 5 times so that it's blended but still nice and thick.

3. After this has been accomplished, pour your salsa into a bowl and serve.

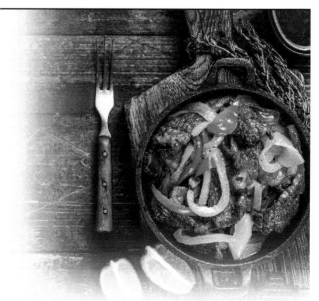

THICK AND CHUNKY SALSA

Preparation Time: 10 minutes

Cooking Time: 55 minutes

Servings: 3

Nutrition:
- calories 114,
- fat 7g,
- fiber 2g,
- carbs 11g,
- protein 8g

Ingredients

½ cup of chopped onion

1 tablespoon of chopped garlic

¼ cup of chopped jalapeño

½ cup of chopped tomatoes

SHEET PAN STEAK FAJITAS

Preparation Time: 10 minutes

Cooking Time: 25 minutes

Servings: 6

Nutrition:
- calories 450,
- fat 26g,
- fiber 2g,
- carbs 4g,

- protein 6g

Ingredients:

For the Steak:
- ½ jalapeño, seeded & finely diced
- ½ tsp. taco seasoning
- 1 ½ lbs. flank steak, sliced
- 1 lime, juiced
- 1 tbsp. extra virgin olive oil
- 1 tsp. garlic powder
- Sea salt & pepper, to taste

For the Veggies:
- ½ tsp. taco seasoning
- 2 lg. onions, thinly sliced
- 2 tbsp. extra virgin olive oil
- 3 lg. bell peppers, thinly sliced
- Sea salt & pepper, to taste

To Serve:
- ½ c. sour cream
- 1 sm. avocado, finely diced
- 2 tbsp. cilantro, fresh & finely chopped
- 8 oz. sharp cheddar cheese, shredded
- 8 small tortillas
- Lime wedges

Direction

1. Preheat the oven to 475° Fahrenheit and line two large baking sheets with non-stick foil.
2. Place the meat into one large mixing bowl, and the vegetables into another.
3. In the mixing bowl with the steak, combine lime juice, taco seasoning, garlic powder, salt, and pepper. Mix completely with tongs or your hands to coat the meat completely in the juice and seasonings.
4. In the mixing bowl with the vegetables, drizzle olive oil, taco seasoning, salt, and pepper. Use hands or tongs to coat completely.
5. Pour half of each bowl onto each baking sheet, then mix thoroughly with your hands so you have two pans filled with identical mixtures.
6. Try to even out the items on the baking pan so they're in one even layer.
7. Bake for 20 minutes or until the steak has reached the desired level of doneness.
8. Broil for 5 minutes to add a little bit of crisp to the meat, then pull sheets out of the oven.
9. Season fajita mixture according to taste, if needed.
10. Serve two fajitas per person!

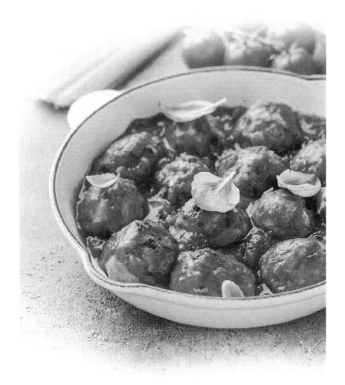

INSTANT POT MEATBALLS

Preparation Time: 10 minutes
Cooking Time: 10 minutes
Servings: 6
Nutrition:
- calories 605,
- fat 23g,
- fiber 2g,
- carbs 8g,
- protein 2g

Ingredients:

- ½ tbsp. balsamic vinegar
- ½ tsp. oregano, dried
- 1 lb. turkey or beef, ground
- 1 lg. egg
- 2 lg. cloves garlic, minced
- 2 tbsp. onion powder
- 15 oz. low-carb tomato sauce
- Sea salt & pepper, to taste

Direction

1. In a large mixing bowl, combine ground meat, onion powder, garlic, oregano, salt, and pepper. Mix completely with your hands.
2. Using a small spoon or scoop, mold the meat into about 30 balls.
3. Pour the tomato sauce into the bottom of the instant pot insert and drop the meatballs into the pot one at a time. It's okay if they overlap!
4. Seal the pressure lock and ensure the pressure valve is sealed. Cook on high for seven minutes.
5. Once the timer beeps, release the pressure completely before opening the lid.
6. Stir to get the tomato sauce all over the meatballs, then serve!

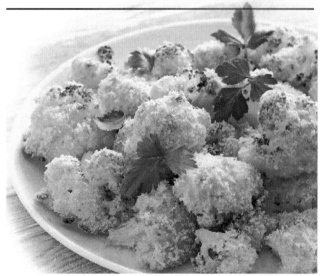

COATED CAULIFLOWER HEAD

Preparation Time: 10 minutes
Cooking Time: 40 minutes
Servings: 6

Nutrition:

- calories 200,
- fat 8g,
- fiber 2g,
- carbs 8g,
- protein 6g

Ingredients:

2-pound cauliflower head
3 tablespoons olive oil
1 tablespoon butter, softened
1 teaspoon ground coriander
1 teaspoon salt
1 egg, whisked
1 teaspoon dried cilantro
1 teaspoon dried oregano
1 teaspoon tahini paste

Directions:

1. Trim cauliflower head if needed.
2. Preheat oven to 350F.
3. In the mixing bowl, mix up together olive oil, softened butter, ground coriander, salt, whisked egg, dried cilantro, dried oregano, and tahini paste.
4. Then brush the cauliflower head with this mixture generously and transfer in the tray.
5. Bake the cauliflower head for 40 minutes.
6. Brush it with the remaining oil mixture every 10 minutes.

CABBAGE CASSEROLE

Preparation Time: 10 minutes
Cooking Time: 55 minutes
Servings: 6
Nutrition:

- calories 273,
- fat 8g,
- fiber 3g,

- carbs 8g,
- protein 9g

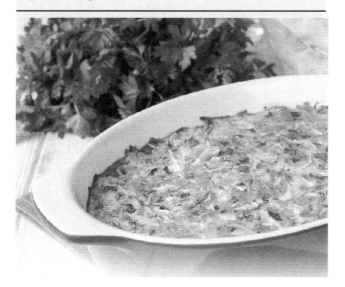

Ingredients:

½ head cabbage

2 scallions, chopped

2 grated carrots

4 tablespoons unsalted butter

2 ounces cream cheese, softened

¼ cup Parmesan cheese, grated

¼ cup fresh cream

½ teaspoon Dijon mustard

2 tablespoons fresh parsley, chopped

Salt and ground black pepper, as required

Directions

1. Preheat your oven to F 350 (180°C).
2. Cut cabbage head into half, lengthwise. Then cut into 4 equal sized wedges.
3. In a pan of boiling water, add cabbage wedges and cook, covered for about 5 minutes.
4. Drain well and arrange cabbage wedges into a small baking dish.
5. In a small pan, melt butter and sauté onions for about 5 minutes.
6. Add the remaining ingredients and stir to combine.
7. Remove from the heat and immediately, place the cheese mixture over cabbage wedges evenly.
8. Bake for about 20 mins.
9. Remove from the oven and let it cool for about 5 minutes before serving.
10. Cut into 3 equal sized portions and serve.

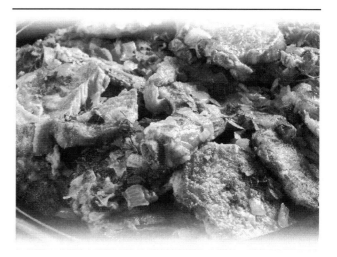

PORK CHOP FEAST

Preparation Time: 10 min

Cooking Time: 50 min

Servings: 3

Nutrition:

- calories 450,
- fat 26g,
- fiber 0g,
- carbs 3g,
- protein 5g

Ingredients

7 pork chops

½ cup of diced onion

¼ cup of diced tomato

1 teaspoon of pepper

1 teaspoon of salt

1 tablespoon of olive oil

Direction

1. Preheat your oven to F. 390
2. Get out a large cooking sheet and grease it with your tablespoon of olive oil.
3. Spread out your 7 pork chops over the cooking sheet.

4. Now add your ½ cup of diced onion and your ¼ cup of diced tomato to the cooking sheet.
5. Season with your teaspoon of salt, and a teaspoon of pepper, and put the cooking sheet into the oven.
6. Cook for 45 minutes.
7. Once cooked, serve immediately.

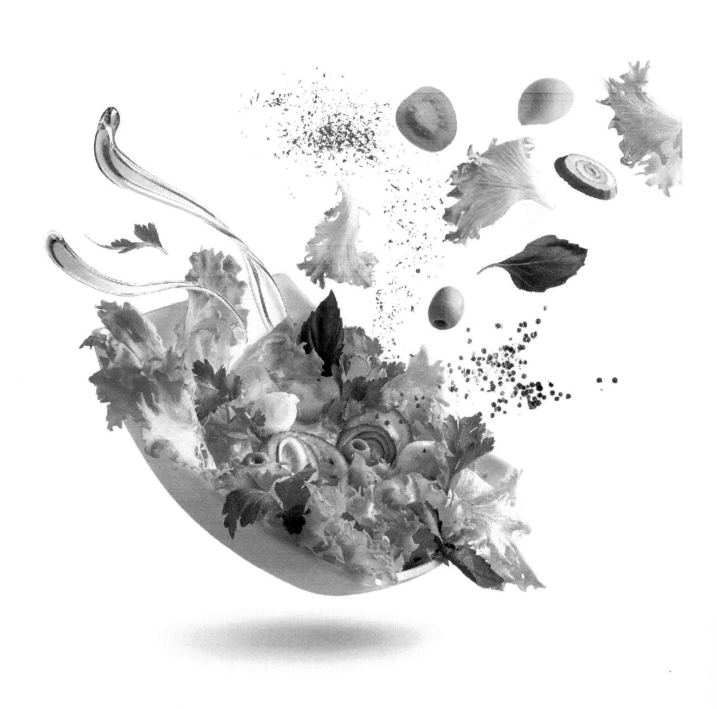

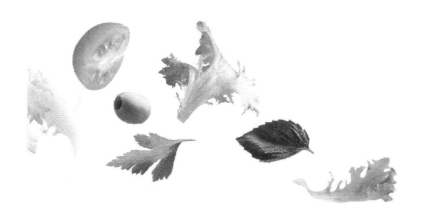

Snacks Sides Salads } for Fasting

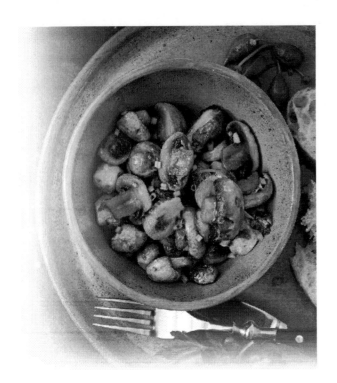

Roasted Brussels Sprouts With Mushrooms and Gorgonzola

Preparation Time: 10 minutes

Cooking Time: 35 minutes

Servings: 4

Nutrition:
- Calories: 149,
- Fat: 11 g
- Carbohydrates: 10 g
- Fiber: 4 g
- Protein: 5 g

Ingredients:

Brussels Sprouts, fresh - 1 pound

Mushrooms, chopped - 1 cup

Olive oil - 1 tablespoon

Extra olive oil to oil the baking tray

Pepper and salt for tasting

Gorgonzola cheese - ¼ cup

(If you prefer not to use the Gorgonzola cheese, you can toss the Brussels sprouts when hot, with 2 tablespoons of butter instead.

Directions:

1. Warm the oven to 350 degrees Fahrenheit or 175 Celsius.
2. Rub a large pan or any vessel you wish to use with a little bit of olive oil. You can use a paper towel or a pastry brush.
3. Cut off the ends of the Brussels sprouts if you need to and then cut then in a lengthwise direction into halves. (Fear not if a few of the leaves come off of them, some may become deliciously crunchy during cooking)
4. Cut the mushrooms.
5. Put your Brussels sprouts as well as the sliced mushrooms inside a bowl, and cover them all with some olive oil, pepper, and salt (be generous).
6. Arrange all of your mushrooms and Brussels sprouts onto your roasting pan in a single layer.
7. Roast this for 30 to 35 minutes, or when they become tender and can be pierced with a fork easily. Stir during cooking if you wish to get a more even browning.
8. Once cooked, toss them with the Gorgonzola Cheese (or butter) before you serve them. Serve them hot.

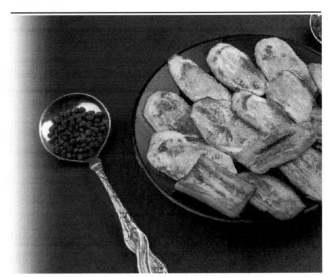

Eggplant Fries

Preparation Time: 10 minutes

Cooking Time: 15 minutes

Servings: 8

Nutrition
- Calories: 212,
- Fat: 15.8 g
- Carbohydrates: 12.1 g
- Protein: 8.6 g

Ingredients:

2 eggs

2 cups almond flour

2 tablespoons coconut oil, spray

2 eggplant, peeled and cut thinly

Salt and pepper

Directions:

1. Preheat your oven to 400 degrees Fahrenheit
2. Take a bowl and mix with salt and black pepper in it
3. Take another bowl and beat eggs until frothy
4. Dip the eggplant pieces into eggs
5. Then coat them with flour mixture
6. Add another layer of flour and egg
7. Then, take a baking sheet and grease with coconut oil on top
8. Bake for about 15 minutes
9. Serve and enjoy.

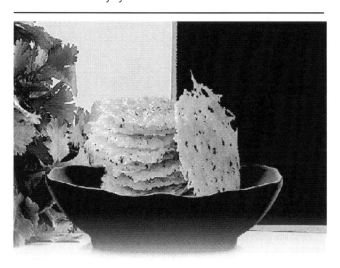

Parmesan Crisps

Preparation Time: 5 minutes
Cooking Time: 25 minutes
Servings: 8

Nutrition:
- Calories: 133,
- Fat: 11 g
- Carbohydrates: 1g
- Protein: 11 g

Ingredients:

1 teaspoon butter

8 ounces parmesan cheese, full fat and shredded

Directions:

1. Preheat your oven to 400 degrees F
2. Put parchment paper on a baking sheet and grease with butter
3. Spoon parmesan into 8 mounds, spreading them apart evenly
4. Flatten them
5. Bake for 5 minutes until browned
6. Let them cool
7. Serve and enjoy.

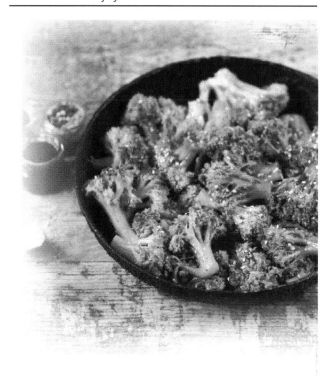

Roasted Broccoli

Preparation Time: 5 minutes
Cooking Time: 20 minutes
Servings: 4

Nutrition:
- Calories: 62,
- Fat: 4 g
- Carbohydrates: 4 g
- Protein: 4 g

Ingredients:

4 cups broccoli florets

1 tablespoon olive oil

Salt and pepper to taste

Directions:

1. Preheat your oven to 400 degrees F
2. Add broccoli in a zip bag alongside oil and shake until coated
3. Add seasoning and shake again
4. Spread broccoli out on the baking sheet, bake for 20 minutes
5. Let it cool and serve.

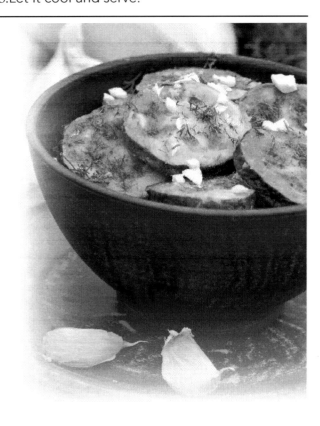

ZUCCHINI CHIPS

Preparation Time: 10 minutes
Cooking Time: 12 minutes
Servings: 4

Nutrition:
- Calories: 106,
- Fat: 8.2 g
- Carbs: 5.2 g
- Protein: 5.1 g
- Fiber 2.1 g

Ingredients:

1 zucchini, thinly sliced

A pinch of sea salt

Black pepper to taste

1 teaspoon thyme, dried

1 egg

1 teaspoon garlic powder

1 cup almond flour

Directions:

1. In a bowl, whisk the egg with a pinch of salt.
2. Put the flour in another bowl and mix it with thyme, black pepper, and garlic powder.
3. Dredge zucchini slices in the egg mix and then in flour.
4. Arrange chips on a lined baking sheet, place in the oven at 450 degrees F and bake for 6 minutes on each side,
5. Serve the zucchini chips as a snack. Enjoy.

PEPPERONI BITES

Preparation Time: 5 minutes
Cooking Time: 10 minutes
Servings: 6 pieces

Nutrition:
- Calories 59,
- Fat 4.5 g
- Fiber 0.1 g
- Carbs 2 g
- Protein 2.5 g

Ingredients:

1/3 cup tomatoes, chopped
½ cup bell peppers, mixed and chopped
3 small peppers halved lengthwise
½ cup tomato sauce
4 ounces almond cheese, cubed
2 tablespoons basil, chopped
Black pepper to taste

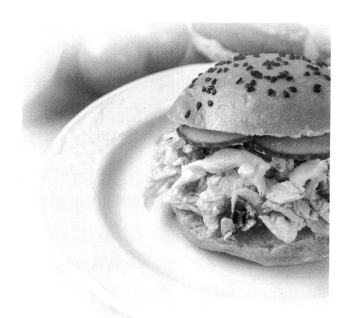

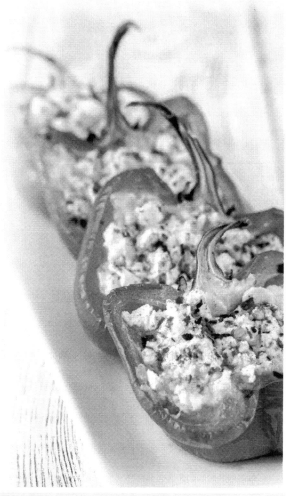

Directions:

1. Divide pepperoni slices into a muffin tray.
2. Divide tomato and bell pepper pieces into the pepperoni cups.
3. Also divide the tomato sauce, basil and almond cheese cubes, sprinkle black pepper at the end, place cups in the oven at 400 degrees F and bake for 10 minutes.
4. Arrange the pepperoni bites on a platter and serve.

HEALTHY SALMON SANDWICH

Preparation Time: 10 minutes
Cooking Time: 10 minutes
Servings: 6

Nutrition:
- Calories 280
- Fats 20g
- Protein 15g
- Carbohydrates 12g

Ingredients

2 salmon fillets (1 Lb)
12 slices of vegan bread
2 eggs
1/2 cup chopped onions
1 tbsp mayonnaise
1 cup gluten-free bread crumbs
2 tsp lemon juice
1/4 tsp garlic salt
1 tbsp chopped fresh parsley
2 tbsp olive oil

Directions

1. Season the salmon using salt and pepper.
2. In a skillet add ½ tbsp of oil and heat it over medium heat.
3. Fry the salmon for 2 minutes on both sides.

4. Let it cool down completely.
5. Remove them bones and mash it finely.
6. In a bowl transfer the salmon. Add the onion, garlic salt, parsley, bread crumbs, mayo and eggs.
7. Pull well with the fork.
8. Let it refrigerate for 30 minutes.
9. In a skillet heat the remaining oil.
10. Fry the slices of bread on both sides.
11. Make sure to fry in batches.
12. Assemble the salad sandwich to taste. Serve hot.

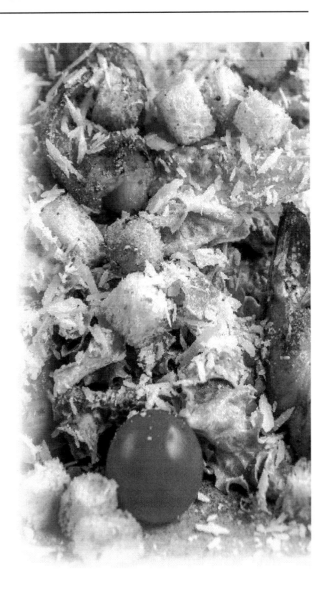

SHRIMP SALAD

Preparation Time: 15 minutes
Cooking Time: 0 minutes
Servings: 8

Nutrition:
- Calories 150
- Carbohydrates 8g
- Fat 8g
- Protein 18g

Ingredients:

1/3 English cucumber, diced

¾ cup of plain yogurt

1 pound of peeled shrimp.

1 tablespoon. Dijon mustard

1 Teaspoon. garlic powder

4 slices of vegan bread cut into cubes.

2 tbsp extra virgin olive oil

2 tbsp. mayo

1 cup of Parmesan

Sea salt and pepper, just enough

Directions:

1. Heat the oven to F 400, line the pan with oiled paper.
2. In a bowl mix the bread and shrimp with oil and garlic.
3. Place on the pan, and bake for 12 min.
4. Let it rest for half an hour.
5. Mix all the ingredients well in a bowl.
6. Serve cold!

BROCCOLI SALAD

Preparation Time: 20 minutes
Cooking Time: 5 minutes
Servings: 6

Nutrition:
- Calories 250
- Carbohydrates 20g
- Fats 16g
- Protein 12g

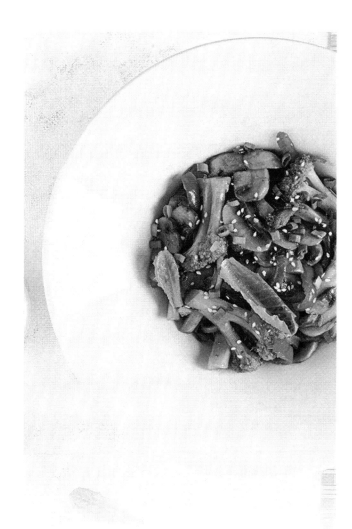

Southwest Chicken Salad

Preparation Time: 15 min

Cooking Time: 15 min

Servings: 8

Nutrition:

- Calories 217
- Carbohydrates 30g
- Fats 9g
- Protein 7g

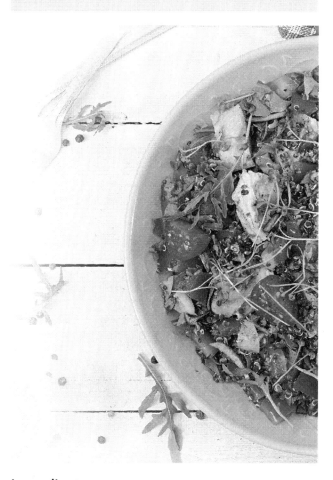

Ingredients:

½ cup of pecans, chopped

1 and a half tablespoons. onion powder

1 pound of broccoli

0.5 pound of mushrooms

1 small pepper, cut into strips

1 tablespoon. apple cider vinegar

2 tbsp of toasted sesame seeds

2 tbsp of extra virgin olive oil

Sea salt and pepper, just enough

Directions:

1. Heat the pan well with oil, and sauté the broccoli and pepperoni.
2. Add the mushrooms and cook until the broccoli is tender.
3. Leave the mixture to rest for 15 min.
4. In a medium bowl, mix all ingredients thoroughly.
5. Serve immediately!

Ingredients:

¼ cup extra virgin olive oil

¼ cup red onion, finely chopped

1 jalapeño, seeded & minced

1 tsp. chili powder

1 tsp. cumin

1 tsp. garlic powder

1 tsp. onion powder

2 bell peppers, diced

2 lg. limes, juiced

2 lb. chicken thighs, cooked and diced

- 2 tbsp. cilantro, finely chopped
- 3 cup quinoa, cooked
- 2 cup arugula
- Sea salt & black pepper, to taste

Directions:

1. In a small bowl, mix chilli powder, lime juice, onion powder, garlic powder, cumin, and cilantro. Mix thoroughly and set aside.
2. In a large mixing bowl, combine all other ingredients and toss until thoroughly combined.
3. Drizzle seasoning mixture over the salad and toss to coat thoroughly.
4. Cover and refrigerate for 30 minutes before serving.

- ¾ cup plain yogurt
- 1 clove garlic, minced
- 1 lg. stalk celery, diced
- 1 tbsp. lemon juice
- 2 small dill pickles, diced
- 24 oz. tuna packed in water, drained
- Sea salt & pepper, to taste

Directions:

1. In a medium bowl, thoroughly mix all ingredients.
2. Chill in the fridge for 12 minutes while covered before serving.
3. Serve chilled!

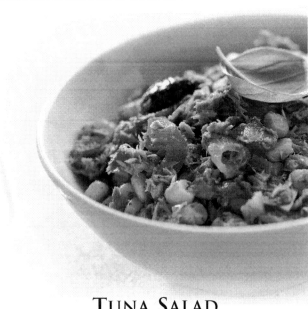

TUNA SALAD

Preparation Time: 15 minutes
Cooking Time: 0 minutes
Servings: 10

Nutrition:
- Calories 152
- Carbohydrates 2g
- Fats 8g
- Protein 18g

Ingredients:
- ¼ cup mayonnaise
- ¼ cup red onion, finely diced

GREEK QUINOA SALAD

Preparation Time: 10 minutes
Cooking Time: 15 minutes
Servings: 4

Nutrition:
- Calories 360
- Carbohydrates 32g
- Fat 23g
- Protein 12g

Ingredients:
- ¼ cup of red onion, finely chopped
- ½ cup of feta cheese crumbles
- ½ cup of finely chopped parsley
- ½ English cucumber, chopped
- 1 cup of quinoa, cooked and cooled
- 1 cup of cooked chickpeas
- 1 lemon, squeezed
- 1 large pepper, chopped
- 10 cherry tomatoes, cut in half
- 1 tablespoon. cumin
- 2 tbsp. extra virgin olive oil

- 20 pitted black olives
- Sea salt and pepper, just enough

Directions:

1. In a medium bowl, mix all ingredients thoroughly.

2. Cover and refrigerate for 15 minutes before serving.

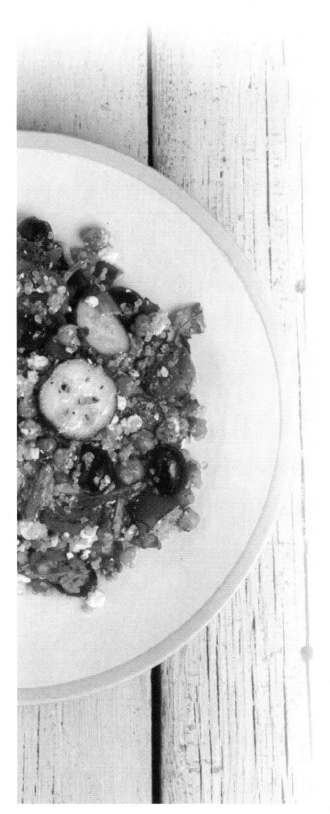

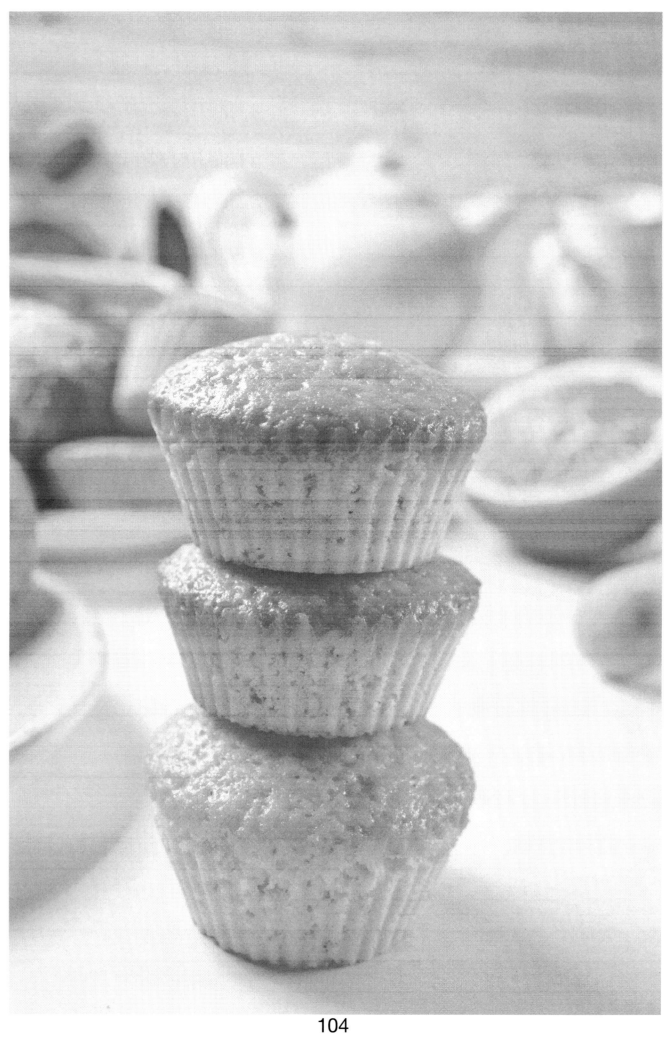

UNIQUE DESSERTS FOR YOUR FAST

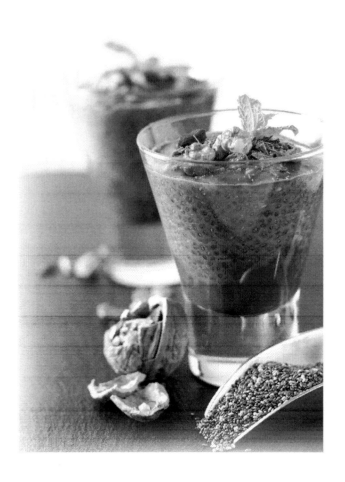

2. Add chia seeds and cocoa powder and mix completely.

3. Allow everything to sit for about 10 minutes before stirring once again, then sealing tightly and storing in the refrigerator overnight.

4. Stir well before eating and enjoy cold!

Mango Lime Chia Pudding

Preparation time: 5 minutes
Cooking time: 30 minutes
Servings: 3

Nutrition:
Calories 156
Protein 11.2g
Carbohydrates 6.2g
Fat 9.7g
Fiber 1.3g

Chocolate Chia Pudding

Cooking Time: 0 minutes
Servings: 1

Nutrition:
- Calories 329
- Carbohydrates 40g
- Fats 14g
- Protein 14g

Ingredients:

¾ cup milk, unsweetened

2 tsp. honey

1 tsp. vanilla extract

4 tbsp. chia seeds

1 tbsp. cocoa powder, unsweetened

Directions:

1. In a glass jar or container, combine all liquid ingredients and mix thoroughly.

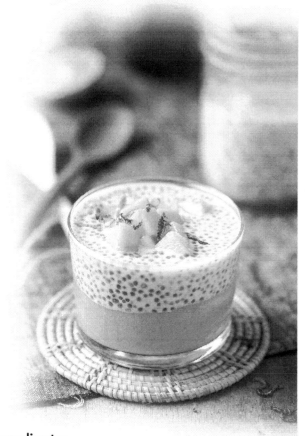

Ingredients:

3 cups fresh or frozen mango chunks

One 15.5-ounce can coconut milk

1 tablespoon lime zest

¼ cup maple syrup

¼ cup freshly squeezed lime juice

¼ cup hemp seeds

1/3 cup chia seeds

Topping options: Approximately 8 cups of any combination of mango, banana, pineapple, or any fruit you'd love with mango and lime. (Banana is a fruit you'd want to wait to add until you are ready to eat the pudding as it browns and gets mushy very quickly once out of its peel)

Directions:

1. Place mango chunks, coconut milk, lime zest, and maple syrup in a blender. Mix until smooth.

2. Add hemp and chia seeds in the blender and stir by hand or blend on low to just combine.

3. This should yield 4 cups of pudding. Portion it as you prefer. One suggestion is to divide into 8 portions, one each in a pint jar, and top with one cup of fresh fruit.

4. Refrigerate pudding until ready to eat, minimum 4 hours to set. The pudding keeps for 5-7 days.

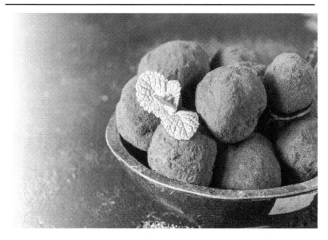

Mint Chocolate Truffle Larabar Bites

Preparation time: 5 minutes
Cooking time: 45 minutes
Servings: 6

Nutrition:
- Calories 202
- Protein 11.7g
- Carbohydrates 29.4g
- Fat 3.8g
- Fiber 3.7g

Ingredients:

1 cup vegan chocolate chips (semi-sweet dark chips are recommended)

10 large Medjool dates

1 ½ cups of raw almonds

¼ cup coconut flour

¼ cup of cocoa powder

¼-1/2 teaspoon peppermint extract

2 tablespoons water

Directions:

1. Pour almonds into a food processor and chop until a fine flour.

2. Add chocolate chips, dates, flour and cocoa, and process again until well combined.

3. Add oil and peppermint extract.

4. Process one more time until the mix starts balling up.

5. Taste a small bit and add more peppermint if you wish. Process again if you do.

6. Remove the blade from the processor and form the dough into balls. Choose whatever size you like, as they do not need to bake and will be good in any portion.

Chocolate Mousse

Preparation time: 5 minutes
Cooking time: 40 minutes
Servings: 6
Nutrition:
- Calories 166
- Protein 9g

- Carbohydrates 2.4g
- Fat 13.5g
- Fiber 0.3g

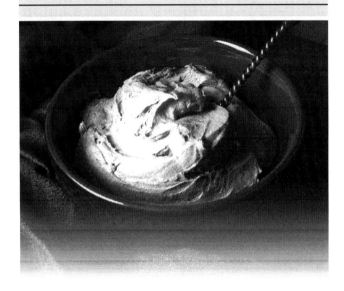

Ingredients:

Cocoa powder – .33 cup

Lakanto monk fruit sweetener – 2 tablespoons

Heavy whipping cream – 1.5 cups

Directions:

1. Place the heavy cream in a bowl and use a hand mixer or stand mixer to beat it on medium speed.

2. Once the cream begins to thicken, add the monk fruit sweetener and cocoa and continue to beat it until stiff peaks form.

3. Serve the mousse immediately or store it in the fridge for up to twenty-four hours before enjoying it. If desired, you can serve it with Lily's stevia-sweetened chocolate for chunks.

NO-BAKE PEANUT BUTTER PIE

Preparation time: 5 minutes

Cooking time: 60 minutes

Servings: 6

Nutrition:

- Calories 166
- Protein 9g
- Carbohydrates 2.4g
- Fat 13.5g
- Fiber 0.3gIngredients:

Almond flour – 1 cup

Butter softened – 2 tablespoons

Vanilla - .5 teaspoon

Lakanto monk fruit sweetener – 1.5 tablespoons

Cocoa powder – 3 tablespoons

Cream cheese softened – 16 ounces

Heavy cream – .75 cup

Vanilla – 2 teaspoons

Swerve confectioner's sweetener - .66 cup

Peanut butter or Sun Butter, unsweetened – .75 cup

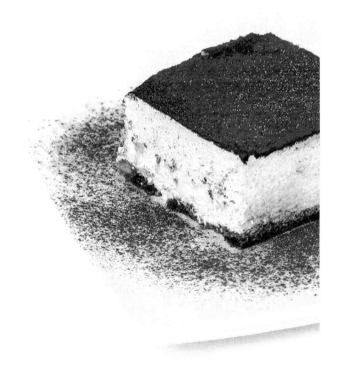

Directions:

1. Combine the almond flour, butter, .5 teaspoon of vanilla, Lakanto sweetener, and cocoa powder in a bowl with a fork until it forms a crumbly mixture. Press this mixture into a nine-inch pie plate and then allow it to chill in the fridge while you prepare the filling.

2. In a large bowl, beat together the cream cheese, peanut butter, confectioners Swerve, and remaining vanilla until light and creamy. Using a spatula scrape down the sides of the bowl before adding in the heavy cream.

3. Beat the filling some more until the heavy cream is incorporated and the mixture is once again light and creamy.

4. Pour the filling into the prepared crust and allow it to chill for two hours before serving. Slice and enjoy.

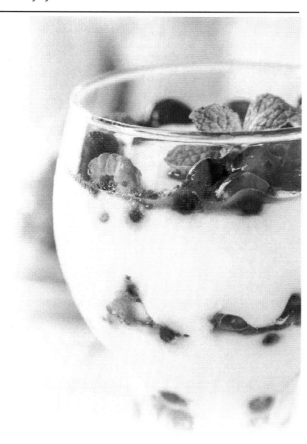

Berries with Ricotta Cream

Preparation time: 5 min
Cooking time: 40 min
Servings: 6
Nutrition:
- Calories 153
- Protein 6.2g
- Carbohydrates 19.2g
- Fat 5.6g
- Fiber 2.6g

Ingredients:
- Ricotta, whole milk – 1.5 cups
- Heavy cream – 2 tablespoons
- Lemon zest – 1.5 teaspoons
- Swerve confectioner's sweetener – .25 cup
- Vanilla extract – 1 teaspoon
- Blackberries - .5 cup
- Raspberries - .5 cup
- Blueberries - .5 cup

Directions:

1. In a large bowl, add all of the ingredients, except for the berries, and whip them together with a hand mixer until completely smooth.

2. Set out four parfait glasses and divide half of the berries between all of them. Top the berries with half of the ricotta mixture, the remaining half of the berries, and lastly, the second half of the ricotta mixture.

3. Serve the parfaits immediately or within the next twenty-four hours.

Easy Chocolate Pudding

Preparation time: 5 minutes
Cooking time: 30 minutes
Servings: 6
Nutrition:
- Calories 231
- Protein 14.9g
- Carbohydrates 3.2g
- Fat 18g
- Fiber 1.1g

Ingredients:

1 ½ cups organic coconut cream from a can

½ cup raw cacao powder

(sifted unsweetened cocoa powder works as well)

6 tablespoons pure maple syrup (may adjust to up

to 8 tablespoons, depending on how sweet you like it)

2 teaspoons pure vanilla extract

Fine-grain sea salt

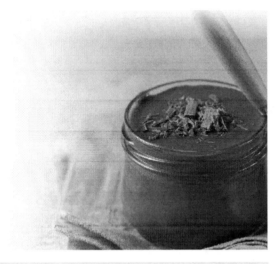

Directions:

1. In a small saucepan over low heat, whisk coconut cream, cacao, and maple syrup until smooth. A smaller whisk my make a smoother mixture. Continue to cook over low/medium for 2 minutes, or until the mixture just starts to come to a boil with small bubbles.

2. Remove from heat. Add salt and vanilla. Stir. Taste and add more maple if you'd like a sweeter pudding.

3. Pour into individual containers/bowls or keep in one larger bowl to set.

4. Cover and refrigerate until set, or overnight for a thick and creamy pudding. Makes 4 servings.

VANILLA MUFFINS

Preparation Time: 5 Minutes
Cooking Time: 2 Minutes
Servings: 4

Nutrition:
- Calories: 75,
- Carbs: 4 g
- Fat: 6 g
- Protein: 3 g

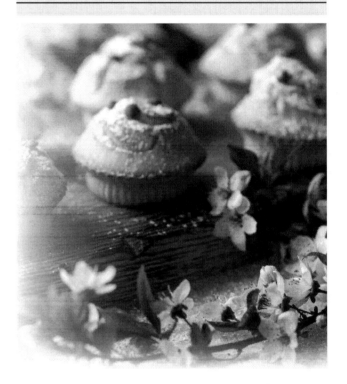

Ingredients:

1 tbsp. Truvia

1 egg, beaten

4 tbsp. coconut flour

1 cup water, for cooking

1 tsp. coconut shred

1 tsp. vanilla extract

¼ tsp. baking powder

Directions:

1. Mix up together all the ingredients and stir well until you get a thick batter

2. Add water in the Ninja Foodi basket. Place the batter into the muffin molds and transfer them on the Ninja Foodi rack.

3. Lower the pressure cooker lid and set Pressure mode High pressure

4. Cook the muffins for 2 minutes. Use the quick pressure release method. Chill the muffins and serve!

Ginger Cookies

Preparation Time: 10 Minutes

Cooking Time: 14 Minutes

Servings: 7

Nutrition:
- Calories: 172,
- Fats: 15.6g,
- Carbohydrates: 4.1g,
- Protein: 4.4 g

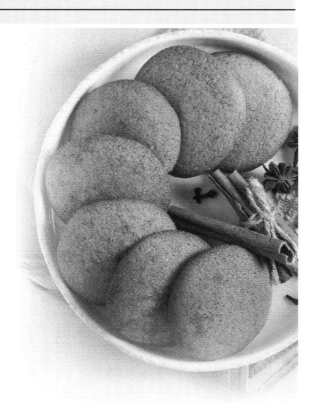

Ingredients:

1 cup almond flour

1 egg

3 tbsp. Erythritol

3 tbsp. heavy cream

3 tbsp. butter

1 tsp. ground ginger

½ tsp. ground cinnamon

½ tsp. baking powder

Directions:

1. Beat the egg in the bowl and whisk it gently. Add baking powder, Erythritol, ground ginger, ground cinnamon, heavy cream, and flour

2. Stir gently and add butter, Knead the non-sticky dough. Roll up the dough with the help of the rolling pin and make the cookies with the help of the cutter.

3. Place the cookies in the basket in one layer and close the lid. Set the Bake mode and cook the cookies for 14 minutes at 350 Degrees F

4. When the cookies are cooked; let them chill well and serve!

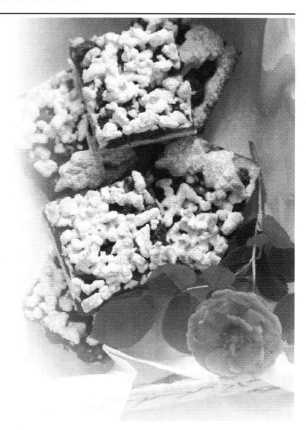

Raspberry Dump Cake

Preparation Time: 10 Minutes

Cooking Time: 30 Minutes

Servings: 10

Nutrition:
- Calories: 107,
- Fats 4.5 g,
- Carbohydrates: 15.1g,
- Protein: 4.3 g

Ingredients:

½ cup raspberries

1 ½ cup coconut flour

1/3 cup almond milk

¼ cup Erythritol

1 egg; whisked

1 tbsp. butter; melted

1 tsp. baking powder

½ tsp. vanilla extract

1 tsp. lemon juice

Directions:

1. Combine together all the dry ingredients. Then add egg, almond milk, and butter

2. Add the vanilla extract and lemon juice. Mix the mixture well. It would be best if you took a liquid batter.

3. Place the cherry layer in the silicone mold. Pour the batter over the cherries

4. Place the mold on the oven rack. Bake the cake for 30 minutes at 350 degrees F.

5. When the cake is cooked; chill it well. Turn upside down and transfer on the serving plate

PUMPKIN PIE

Preparation Time: 10 Minutes

Cooking Time: 25 Minutes

Servings: 6

Nutrition:
- Calories: 127,
- Fat: 6.6g,
- Carbohydrates: 14.2 g,
- Protein: 3.8 g

Ingredients:

1 cup coconut flour

¼ cup heavy cream

1 egg; whisked

1 tbsp. butter

2 tbsp. liquid stevia

1 tbsp. pumpkin puree

1 tsp. apple cider vinegar

1 tsp. Pumpkin spices

½ tsp. baking powder

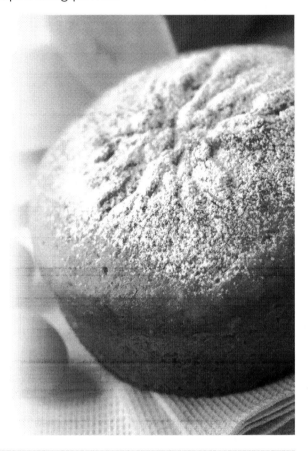

Directions:

1. Melt the butter and combine it together with the heavy cream, apple cider vinegar, liquid stevia, egg, and baking powder

2. Add pumpkin puree and coconut flour. Now, add pumpkin spices and stir the batter until smooth.

3. Pour the batter in Ninja Foodi basket and lower the air fryer lid

4. Set the "Bake" mode 360 Degrees F. Cook the pie for 25 minutes. When the time is over; let the pie chill till the room temperature.

AVOCADO MOUSSE

Preparation Time: 2 Minutes

Cooking Time: 10 Minutes

Servings: 7

Nutrition:
- Calories: 144,
- Fats: 13.9 g,
- Carbohydrates: 10.5 g,
- Protein: 1.3 g

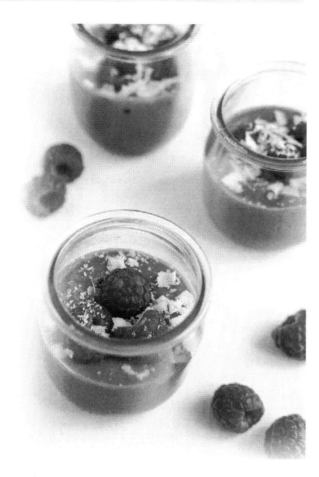

Ingredients:

2 avocados, peeled, cored

3 tbsp. Erythritol

1/3 cup heavy cream

1 tsp. butter

1 tsp. vanilla extract

1 tsp. of cocoa powder

Directions:

1. Preheat Ninja Foodi at "Sauté" mode for 5 minutes. Meanwhile, mash the avocado until smooth and mix it up with Erythritol

2. Place the butter in the pot and melt. Add mashed avocado mixture and stir well.

3. Add cocoa powder and stir until homogenous. Sauté the mixture for 3 minutes

4. Meanwhile, whisk the heavy cream on high speed for 2 minutes. Transfer the cooked avocado mash in the bowl and chill in ice water.

5. When the avocado mash reaches room temperature; add whisked heavy cream and vanilla extract. Stir gently to get white-chocolate swirls

6. Transfer the mousse into small cups and chill for 4 hours in the fridge.

7. Before serving, you can add some fresh fruit.

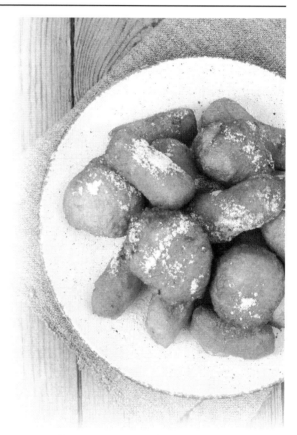

Almond Bites

Preparation Time: 10 Minutes

Cooking Time: 14 Minutes

Servings: 5

Nutrition:
- Calories: 118,
- Fats: 11.5 g,
- Carbohydrates: 2.4 g,
- Protein: 2.7 g

Ingredients:
- 1 cup almond flour

- ¼ cup almond milk
- 1 egg; whisked
- 2 tbsp. butter
- 1 tbsp. coconut flakes
- ½ tsp. baking powder
- ½ tsp. apple cider vinegar
- ½ tsp. vanilla extract

Directions:

1. Mix up together the whisked egg, almond milk, apple cider vinegar, baking powder, vanilla extract, and butter
2. Stir the mixture and add almond flour and coconut flakes. Knead the dough.
3. If the dough is sticky, add more almond flour. Make medium balls from the dough and place them on the wire rack on a lined baking sheet.
4. Bake the cake in the preheated oven for 12 minutes at 360 degrees F.
5. Check if the dessert is cooked; and cook for 2 minutes more for a crunchy crust

Ingredients:

Bosc pears, ripe - 4

Marsala wine - 1½ cups

Directions:

1. Preheat oven to 450°F.
2. Place pears upright in a baking dish and pour the marsala wine over them. Bake the pears for 20 minutes. Add water or more marsala if the dish starts to get dry.
3. Baste the pears with the liquid in the dish and bake 20 minutes more.
4. Baste the pears again and bake longer until a knife inserted in a pear goes in easily.
5. Take out the pears and baste them several times as they cool.
6. Serve at room temperature to taste with a little whipped cream and a sprinkle of cinnamon.

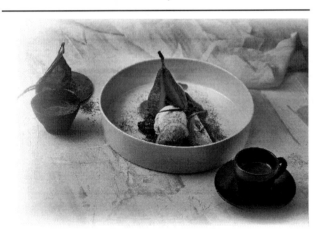

OVEN-ROASTED PEARS

Preparation Time: 6 minutes;

Cooking Time: 55 minutes;

Servings: 4

Nutrition:
- Calories: 217,
- Fat: 0.5g,
- Protein: 1g,
- Carbs: 31g

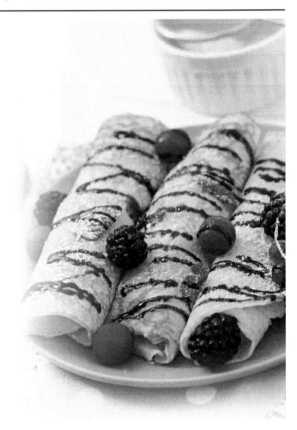

ALMOND FLOUR CREPES

Preparation Time: 5 minutes

Cooking Time: 5 minute

Servings: 4

Nutrition:
- Calories: 170
- Fat: 12g
- Carbohydrates: 8g
- Protein: 12g

Ingredients

6 large eggs, room temperature

1 cup blanched almond flour

1 tsp almond or vanilla extract

3 tbsp chocolate sauce for serving

1/2 Fresh mixed berries, for serving

2 tbsp natural honey

1 cup almond milk

Directions:

1. In a bowl, beat the eggs, almond flour and 1/3 cup almond milk, pear to obtain a homogeneous and smooth mixture.

2. Place an 8-inch non-stick skillet over medium heat, lightly sprinkling with cooking oil spray.

3. Ladle the crepe batter into the pan, tilting it in a circular motion to evenly coat the cooking surface.

4. Cook the crepe for 2 minutes until the edges turn golden and lift easily from the pan.

5. Loosen with a spatula and flip, cooking the other side for 1-2 minutes, until golden brown. Repeat with the remaining batter.

6. When serving, sprinkle each crepe with honey diluted with almond milk and fresh berries.

CARROT CAKE

Preparation Time: 15 Minutes

Cooking Time: 25 Minutes

Servings: 8

Nutrition:
- Calories: 135,
- Fat: 8g,
- Carbohydrates: 18 g,
- Protein: 5 g

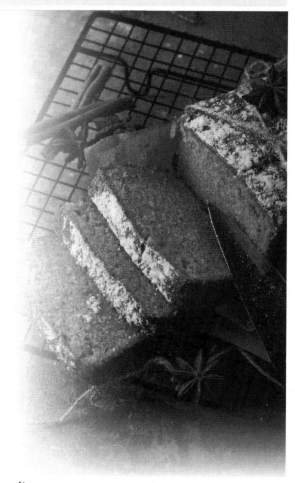

Ingredients:

1.5 cups almond flour

¼ cup heavy cream

1/2 cup erythritol

5 tablespoon butter, softened

4 egg; whisked

2 teaspoon ground cinnamon

1/2 teaspoon ground ginger

1 cup carrot, finely grated

1 tsp. apple cider vinegar

½ tsp. baking powder

Directions:

1. Preheat the oven to F 350.

2. Line a plum-cake mold with parchment paper and set it aside.

3. In a bowl, whisk the butter and erythritol together until light in color.

4. Beat the eggs into the butter mixture until incorporated.

5. Add the spices and baking powder, then whisk to combine.

6. Add the almond flour and mix well again.

7. Add the grated carrot and incorporate it into the batter.

8. Pour the batter into the pan and roll out the top to evenly distribute the batter. Cook for 18-25 minutes or until an inserted toothpick is clean.

9. Serve at room temperature.

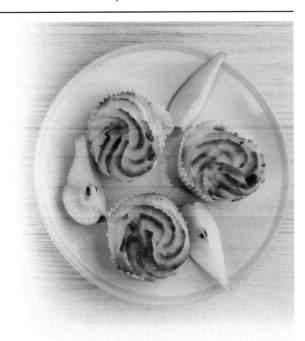

Almond flour pear muffin

Preparation Time: 15 Minutes

Cooking Time: 25 Minutes

Servings: 8

Nutrition:
- Calories: 60,
- Fat: 3.9 g,
- Carbohydrates: 10 g,
- Protein 4.5 g

Ingredients:

1 cups almond flour

1 teaspoons baking powder

1/2 teaspoon baking soda

1/4 teaspoon sea salt

2 large eggs

1 tablespoons vanilla extract

1 tablespoon lemon zest

1 cup lightly packed brown sugar

8 tablespoons unsalted butter, melted

1 cup unsweetened applesauce or pear sauce

1 to 2 ripe pears, thinly sliced, for muffin tops

2 tablespoons vanilla sugar for muffin tops

Directions:

1. Preheat oven to 400 degrees F. Line molds with muffin paper cups.

2. In a bowl, beat the flour, baking powder, baking soda, nutmeg, and salt. In another bowl, beat the eggs, vanilla extract, lemon zest, and brown sugar until smooth. Stir in the melted butter, a little at a time, beating until you get a creamy mixture.

3. Mix the two compounds with a spatula until they are well combined.

4. Divide the batter between the muffin tins. Sprinkle the tops with a sprinkle of vanilla sugar.

5. Bake the muffins until leavened and golden, about 20 minutes. Remove from the oven and leave to cool in the pan for 5 minutes.

Coconut Macaroon Cookies

Preparation Time: 5 Minutes

Cooking Time: 15 Minutes

Servings: 18

Nutrition:
- Calories: 150,
- Fat: 7 g,
- Carbohydrates: 20 g,
- Protein 2 g

Ingredients:

5 cups coconut (finely shredded, unsweetened)

1 1/2 cup brown sugar

Pinch of salt

4 large egg whites (lightly beaten)

1 teaspoon pure vanilla extract

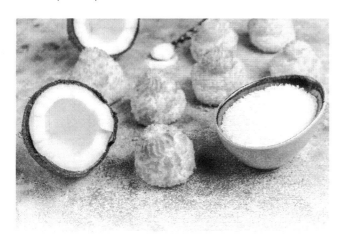

Directions:

1. Preheat the oven to 350 F. Line 2 large baking sheets with parchment paper.
2. In a large mixing bowl, mix the coconut, sugar, and salt. Add the egg whites and vanilla extract, mixing until well combined.
3. Using your hands, form the mixture into small 1 1/2 to 2 tablespoon mounds, transferring each to the prepared baking sheets as you work.
4. Bake until just the cookies' peaks is light golden brown, about 12 to 15 minutes, turning the pan halfway through to ensure even baking.
5. Allow the cookies to cool completely on a wire cooling rack. Serve at room temperature.

ALMOND FLOUR MUFFINS

Preparation Time: 15 minutes
Cooking Time: 30 minutes
Servings: 8
Nutrition:

- Calories: 75,
- Carbs: 4 g
- Fat: 6 g
- Protein: 3 g

Ingredients:

1/3 cup of pumpkin puree

3 eggs

2 tablespoons agave nectar

2 tablespoons coconut oil

1 teaspoon vanilla extract

1 teaspoon white vinegar

1 cup chopped fruits

1 teaspoon baking soda

½ teaspoon salt

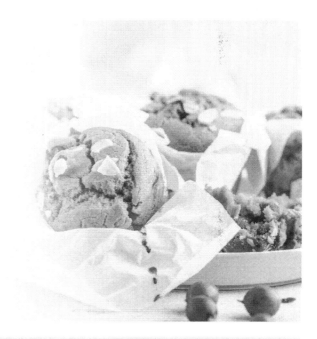

Directions:

1. Preheat the oven to 350°F.
2. Line the muffin tin with paper liners
3. In the first mixing bowl, whisk the almond flour, salt, and baking soda.
4. In the second mixing bowl, whisk the pumpkin puree, eggs, coconut oil, agave nectar, vanilla extract, and vinegar.
5. Now add this puree mix of the second bowl to the first bowl and blend everything well.
6. Add the chopped fruits to the blend.

7. Pour the mixture to the muffin cups in your pan.
8. Bake for 15-20 minutes. Ensure that the contents have set in the center, and a golden-brown lining has started to appear at the edges.
9. Transfer the muffins to a cooling rack and let it cool completely.

Directions:
1. Blend almonds in a food processor until a flour is formed. Add the water and dates to the flour and continue to process until thoroughly combined. You may need to stop intermittently to scrape down the sides of the bowl.
2. Add cocoa and protein to the processor and continue to process until well combined. You may need to stop intermittently to scrape down the sides of the bowl.
3. Pull the blade out of the processor (carefully!) and use your spatula to gather all of the dough in one place inside the processor container.
4. On a plate or in a large, shallow dish, spread the coconut flakes.
5. Scoop out a little bit of the dough at a time using a spoon, and roll it into balls, then move each one in the coconut flakes.
6. Refrigerate for at least 30 min before enjoying.

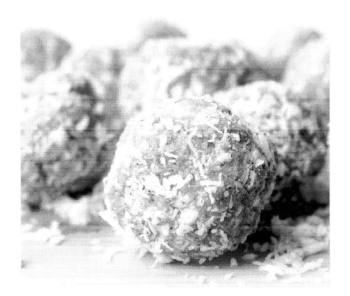

Coconut Protein Balls

Preparation Time: 20 minutes
Cooking Time: 0 minutes
Servings: 27

Nutrition
- Calories 108
- Carbohydrates 16g
- Fats 4g
- Protein 5g

Ingredients:
- ¼ cup dark chocolate chips
- ½ cup coconut flakes, unsweetened
- ½ cup water
- 1 ½ cup almonds, raw & unsalted
- 2 tbsp. cocoa powder, unsweetened
- 3 cup Medjool dates, pitted
- 4 scoops whey protein powder, unsweetened

Blueberry Muffins

Preparation Time: 5 minutes
Cooking Time: 25 minutes
Servings: 12

Nutrition
- Calories 329
- Carbohydrates 40g
- Fats 14g
- Protein 14g

Ingredients:
½ tsp. baking soda
¼ cup vegetable oil
¼ tsp. salt
1 ½ cup blueberries, frozen
1 cup applesauce, unsweetened

1 tsp. vanilla extract

1/3 cup honey

2 cup whole wheat flour

1 tsp. cinnamon

2 large eggs, beaten

2 tsp. baking powder

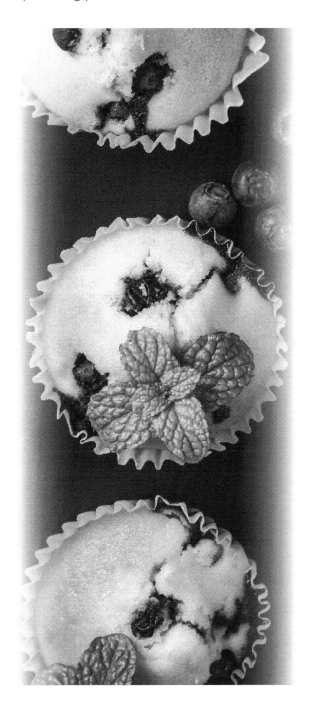

powder in a bowl. Whisk until thoroughly combined, ensuring that there are no lumps of baking powder or soda.

3. Add flour to the batter and whisk until just combined.

4. Add blueberries and mix.

5. Fill the muffin tins and bake for 22-25 minutes or until a toothpick inserted into the middle of the middlemost muffin becomes clean.

6. Let cool for 30 minutes before transferring to a cooling rack to cool completely.

7. Serve and enjoy!

Low-carb waffles

Preparation time: 10 minutes

Cooking time: 20 minutes

Servings: 4

Nutrition:

- calories 200,
- fat 8g,
- fiber 2g,
- carbs 8g,
- protein 6g

Ingredients

6 eggs

2 mashed bananas

2 tsp unsweetened almond butter

3 tsp Quinoa flour

1/4 tsp Salt

1/2 tsp Cinnamon powder

1/2 tsp Olive oil extra virgin.

1/2 tsp Coconut butter.

Sliced quarter banana

1/2 tsp Walnuts chopped.

1 tbsp Maple syrup.

Directions:

1. Preheat oven to 350° Fahrenheit and line a muffin tin with paper liners.

2. Combine eggs, apple sauce, honey, oil, vanilla extract, cinnamon, baking soda, salt, and baking

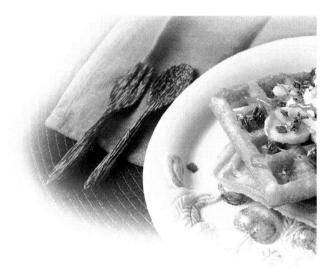

Directions

1. Plug in the waffle maker and let it heat up
2. Get a mixing container and in it mix the bananas mashed, eggs, quinoa flour, cinnamon, unsweetened almond butter, and salt until you get a smooth mixture.
3. When the waffle maker is hot enough, use the extra virgin olive oil to grease it.
4. Divide the waffle mixture into three portions and cook each until it is ready. Remove and do the same for the remaining mixture as well.
5. When cooled off, top the waffles with the remaining almond butter, quarter sliced bananas, and walnuts chopped maple syrup, and coconut butter.

ALMOND APPLE SPICE MUFFINS

Preparation Time: 10 minutes
Cooking Time: 55 minutes
Servings: 5
Nutrition:
- calories 484,
- fat 31g,
- fiber 2g,
- carbs 8g,
- protein 40g

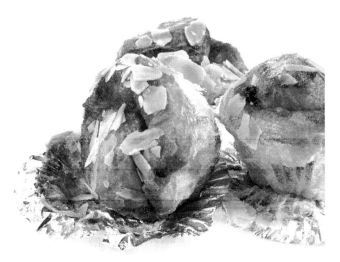

Ingredients
- Butter, half stick
- Almond meal, 2 cups
- Eggs, 4 larges
- Unsweetened applesauce 1 cup
- Cinnamon 1 tbsp.
- Protein powder of Vanilla 4 scoops
- All spice 1 tsp
- Cloves 1 tsp.
- Baking powder 2 tsp

Direction

1. Settle the oven to 350 degrees F. Melt the butter in the microwave at low heat for almost 30 seconds in a small microwave-secure bowl.
2. In a large tub, combine the rest of the ingredients thoroughly with the butter. Sprinkle two muffin tins with a nonstick cooking spray or using a cupcake lining.
3. Pour the mixture into the muffin tins, ensuring that it is not overfilled (about three-fourths full). We expect to prepare ten muffins.
4. Position a tray in the oven and bake for 12 minutes. Make sure you do not overcook

because the muffins will be too hard. When it finishes, take out the first utensil from the oven and bake the second tin likewise.

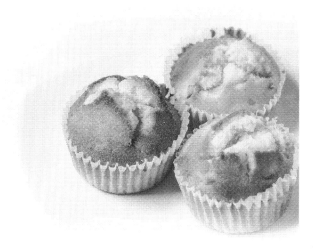

Vegan Coconut Kefir Banana Muffins

Preparation Time: 5 minutes
Cooking Time: 60 minutes
Servings: 6

Nutrition:
- calories 212,
- fat 7g,
- fiber 2g,
- carbs 35g,
- protein 2g

Ingredients
- All-purpose flour, one and a half cups
- Crushed sugar, 1 cup
- Unsweetened shredded coconut 250 mL
- Baking soda 2 teaspoon
- Baking powder 1 teaspoon
- Salt 1/2 tsp
- Ripe mashed bananas 2
- Coconut milk, dairy-free one and a half cups
- Pure Vanilla extract 1 tsp
- Liquid Coconut Oil, one-fourth cup

Direction
1. Settle the oven to 180 ° C. Sprinkle cooking spray on muffin tin. Put it aside.
2. In a big bowl, whisk together sugar, flour, baking powder, shredded coconut, salt, and baking soda. Place it aside.
3. In a separate big cup, mix bananas, vanilla, and coconut oil. Put the flour and mix, whisk until there are no white stripes left.
4. Add mixture in muffin pot. Keep baking till the upper parts are golden and the spatula put in the middle comes out clear, around 30 minutes. Allow chilling the muffin tin for 15 minutes.

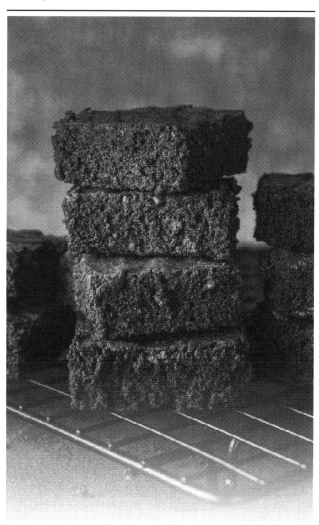

Low - Carb Brownies

Preparation Time: 10 minutes
Cooking Time: 20 minutes
Servings: 16

Nutrition:
- Calories 107
- Fats 10g

- Carbohydrates 5.7g
- Protein 2.5g

Ingredients:

- 7 tablespoons Coconut oil, melted
- 6 tablespoons Plant-Based sweetener
- 1 Large egg
- 2 Egg yolk
- 1/2 tsp Mint extract
- 5 ounces Sugar-free dark chocolate
- ¼ cup Plant-based chocolate protein powder
- 1 tsp Baking soda
- ¼ tsp Sea salt
- 2 tbsp vanilla almond milk, Unsweetened

Directions:

1. Start by preheating the oven to 350°F and then take an 8x8 inch pan and line it with parchment paper, being sure to leave some extra sticking up to use later to help you get them out of the pan after they are cooked.

2. Into a medium-sized vessel, use a hand mixer, and blend 5 Tablespoons of the coconut oil (save the rest for later), as well as the egg, Erythritol, egg yolks, and the mint extract all together for 1 minute. After this minute, the mixture will become a lighter yellow hue.

CONCLUSION

Intermittent fasting is not a new Direction of dieting. In fact, people have been doing it since the beginning of time. Certain fasts such as the Ramadan fast, Lent, etc. have been practiced since ancient times. These fasts, though based on beliefs and religions, are still forms of intermittent fasts and have similar positive effects as well. Intermittent fasting basically means eating at particular times during the day and fasting for the remaining time. So, for example, if you have your breakfast at 8:00 a.m., you are supposed to fast until 8:00 p.m. The fasting period allows your body a resting period and leads to weight loss, glucose regulation and various other benefits.

There exist a variety of intermittent fasts. Some of them are easy to do while some are quite difficult for beginners. Regardless of the ease of an intermittent fast, it can still be one of the most difficult things you ever do if you have never fasted before. You need to regulate your diet cycle, which can be quite a task for many. Yet, it can't be compared to the grueling fact that you need to go 'hungry' for 8-10-12 or even more hours of the day. Eating one or two meals per day and going 'hungry' for the rest is especially difficult for people who are busy and are often accustomed to eating anything they find whenever they get the time. Such people avoid doing intermittent fasting because they believe that they cannot stick to the diet or will go hungry.

Since intermittent fasting is not limiting in what you can eat, there is a wide variety to choose from. All you should have in mind is the number of calories you are consuming per meal. Meals that have low carbohydrate content are ideal because they, in turn, have low caloric content as well. Having more lean meats, fruits, and vegetables is ideal together with grains too.

Learn as many recipes as possible and prepare them for yourself in order to better manage the ingredients being used. You can even do a meal prep whereby you take one day to prepare the meals you wish to eat during the coming one week. This means even when you are too busy or too tired to cook, all you have to do is get your prepped meal, warm it, and enjoy a healthy meal. One reason to go for fast food is that it is readily available. Preparing your meals in advance can help you cover this.

Before making dietary changes, it is always best to consult with a qualified healthcare professional, even if you just change the timing when you eat food. They can help you figure out if intermittent fasting would be good for you. This is particularly important for long-term fasts where there may be vitamin and mineral depletion. It's important to understand how incredibly smart our bodies are. The body will increase appetite and the number of calories consumed at the next meal if food is limited at one meal, and even slow down the metabolism to match calorie consumption. Further, intermittent fasting has many potential health benefits, but it should not be concluded that, if strictly followed, huge weight loss is assured, and disease creation or progression avoided. It is a useful tool, but it may require other tools to help achieve and maintain optimal health.

Thank you

Made in the USA
Monee, IL
30 April 2021